New Practice-based Learning in the Allied Health Professions

This innovative book presents a new, comprehensive overview of the range of approaches available for delivering practice-based learning in allied health professions.

With a strong educational focus, the book provides actionable strategies to deliver positive placement experiences for students, educators and universities alike. It features international contributions from both educators and practitioners, and brings together new models and ideas for the first time. These include evidence-informed evaluation of long-arm supervision, peer-assisted learning and technology-assisted placements, and simulated and interprofessional placements. Each chapter is also supported by case studies which illustrate the dynamics of each model, alongside guidance to students in preparing themselves beforehand. Both practical and timely, the book recognises the critical role that practice educators play in planning, designing, supporting, delivering and assessing practice-based learning experiences – whether in clinical, research or leadership contexts.

Offering a key resource to shape high-quality, impactful placements in allied health education, it will be essential reading for educators, practitioners and students across the allied health professions.

Emma Green is a senior lecturer in occupational therapy, lead for occupational therapy practice-based learning in the Department of Allied Health Professions, Glasgow Caledonian University.

Anita Volkert is a senior lecturer in occupational therapy and the allied health practice placements lead at Glasgow Caledonian University.

Eric Nkansah Opoku is a lecturer in occupational therapy and the departmental lead for equality, diversity and inclusion in the Department of Allied Health Professions at Glasgow Caledonian University.

Katrina Bannigan is a research assistant in the Department of Mental Wellbeing, University of Glasgow.

New Practice-based Learning in the Allied Health Professions

A Toolkit for Innovation and Excellence

EDITED BY EMMA GREEN,
ANITA VOLKERT,
ERIC NKANSAH OPOKU
AND KATRINA BANNIGAN

Routledge
Taylor & Francis Group

LONDON AND NEW YORK

Designed cover image: Getty Images

First published 2026
by Routledge
4 Park Square, Milton Park, Abingdon, Oxon OX14 4RN

and by Routledge
605 Third Avenue, New York, NY 10158

Routledge is an imprint of the Taylor & Francis Group, an informa business

British Library Cataloguing-in-Publication Data
A catalogue record for this book is available from the British Library

ISBN: 978-1-032-53381-0 (hbk)
ISBN: 978-1-032-53382-7 (pbk)
ISBN: 978-1-003-41176-5 (ebk)

DOI: 10.4324/9781003411765

Typeset in Vectora LH
by Apex CoVantage, LLC

Contents

Contributors

CHAPTER AUTHORS

Isaac Amanquarnor, senior lecturer, Division of Occupational Therapy, University of West of England (UK)

Katrina Bannigan, research assistant in the Department of Mental Wellbeing, University of Glasgow (UK)

Jennie Brentnall, senior lecturer, The University of Sydney (Australia)

Kerryn Dillon, Chief People Officer, I-Med Radiology Network (Australia)

Rosemary Xorlanyo Doe-Asinyo, lecturer (education), Division of Occupational Therapy, Brunel University, London (UK)

Lisa Forrest, senior lecturer in occupational therapy, Glasgow Caledonian University (UK)

Roshan Galvaan, professor of occupational therapy and Head of the Department of Health and Rehabilitation Sciences, University of Cape Town (South Africa)

Pragashnie Govender, full professor of occupational therapy in the College of Health Sciences, University of KwaZulu-Natal, Durban (South Africa)

Emma Green, senior lecturer in occupational therapy, Glasgow Caledonian University (UK)

Rowenna Harrison, lecturer in occupational therapy, Glasgow Caledonian University (UK)

Belinda Judd, senior lecturer, University of Sydney (Australia)

Carolyn McDonald is the Chief Allied Health Professions Officer for Scotland (CAHPO) appointed in January 2020 and an occupational therapist by background.

Deshini Naidoo, associate professor of occupational therapy in the College of Health Sciences, University of KwaZulu-Natal, Durban (South Africa).

Eric Nkansah Opoku, lecturer, at Glasgow Caledonian University (UK)

Merrolee Penman, associate professor, teaching and research academic, Curtin University (Australia)

Liesl Peters, senior lecturer, Department of Health and Rehabilitation Sciences, University of Cape Town (South Africa)

Susan Pride, senior occupational therapist, NHS Lanarkshire (UK)

Sandra Robertson, professional lead and senior lecturer in occupational therapy, Glasgow Caledonian University (UK)

Jou Yin Teoh, honorary senior lecturer – life sciences, Division of Occupational Therapy, Brunel University, London (UK)

Jennifer Turnbull, lecturer, Department of Podiatry and Radiography, Glasgow Caledonian University (UK)

Anita Volkert, senior lecturer in occupational therapy, Glasgow Caledonian University (UK)

Claudine Wallace, senior lecturer in orthoptics, Glasgow Caledonian University (UK)

CASE STUDY CONTRIBUTORS

Kathrine Denton, occupational therapist advanced practitioner, Occupational Therapy – Children and Young people, NHS Lanarkshire (UK).

Ashleigh Graham, senior practitioner in Clinical Research (weight management dietitian), NHS Scotland.

Esther May, professor and pro vice chancellor – Teaching and Learning, University of South Australia (Australia).

Catherine McQuade, MSK podiatrist, Western Isles Hospital, Stornoway NHS, Western Isles (UK).

Sarah Miles, clinical educator, Occupational Therapy & Clinical Education team leader; Allied Health, University Centre for Rural Health, The University of Sydney (Australia)

Laura O'Halloran, AHP practice education lead, NHS Western Isles/Senior Educator NHS Education for Scotland (UK).

Samantha Paterson, lecturer in paramedicine, Glasgow Caledonian University, Scotland (UK)

Janet Thompson, team lead, advanced practitioner occupational therapist, Maryhill Health Centre, NHS Moray (UK)

Monica Vasquez, senior occupational therapist, clinical educator, Liverpool Hospital, South Western Sydney Local Health District (Australia)

Figures

Tables

Preface

This book is written for those who are passionate about shaping the future workforce of their profession. Practice-based learning as part of education programmes brings together academic theory and workplace practice to develop skills and competences for our students – and through their insights, challenges and perspectives, we also learn and grow.

Reflecting on my own journey as a student, I am reminded about how valuable my practice-based learning experience was, and I have a personal appreciation of the power of learning in context. The richness of those placements, the teaching and mentorship I received and the real-world application of academic learning to the clinical environment were key to developing my clinical skills and also contributed to shaping my values and professional identity.

Today, the landscape of health and social care continues to evolve – and so, too, must the practice-based learning opportunities, using evidence to develop new models. Hospitals and clinical settings remain vital but we must also embrace contemporary community-based models where people live their lives – not just where they receive treatment. This broader view allows students to understand health and their role in its widest sense – as a lived, social experience influenced by environment, relationships and culture.

We are all individuals and it is essential to recognise that every individual brings their own unique background, identity and lived experience into the learning environment – and this is as true for our students as it is for our colleagues and patients.

As educators and practitioners, we have a responsibility to create spaces where all students feel seen, heard and valued – and embedding principles of equality, diversity and belonging into our teaching and supervision is not an optional add-on; it is fundamental to supporting learning, fostering professional growth and ensuring that students have the opportunity to thrive.

When we create thoughtful, inclusive and encouraging placements, we do not just support student growth; we nurture the future of our professions.

Interprofessional learning remains a cornerstone of high-quality practice-based education. Collaborating across professional boundaries not only reflects the reality of modern healthcare but also enriches students' understanding of their own roles within and across the broader system. Learning with others encourages mutual respect, communication and a person-centred approach to care.

The rapid integration of new technologies, including clinical simulation, robotics and artificial intelligence (AI) is transforming the way we deliver services and educate future practitioners. From AI-assisted diagnostics to robotic rehabilitation tools, these innovations are reshaping practice and creating new learning opportunities. It is essential for our students to engage with these developments to acquire the confidence and critical thinking required to navigate a health and social care landscape that is increasingly digital, data-driven and interdisciplinary.

As teachers, mentors and professional role models, we must be mindful that the students we support today are our colleagues tomorrow. They are the future of our professions. Investing in their learning through meaningful, inclusive and contextually relevant placements is not only an educational responsibility but a professional one. The responsibility to support student education in practice belongs to all of us, reflecting our commitment to the continued growth and excellence of all of our professions.

Professor Carolyn McDonald
Chief Allied Health Professions Officer (Scotland)

Chapter 1

Introduction

Context and rationale for contemporary approaches to practice-based learning

Emma Green and Anita Volkert

CHAPTER OVERVIEW

This book brings together for the first time innovative approaches to delivering practice-based learning in the allied health professions. It presents a wide portfolio of placement models, providing not only a comprehensive overview but also insights into the broader context of how to successfully implement practice-based learning for pre-registration learners in allied health. The book has a strong educational focus aimed to support the design and implementation of practical, real-world placement models. The essence of the book is to provide actionable strategies to deliver good placement experiences for learners, practice educators and universities alike. The book draws on evidence-based research to guide the design and implementation of these placement models. To make these concepts tangible, the book includes real-world examples from a variety of allied health pre-registration programmes across the globe, demonstrating how these models can be applied effectively in practice. Whether you are an educator, a practitioner or a learner, this book is a vital tool for shaping high-quality, impactful placements in allied health education.

In this introductory chapter, we will lay the foundation by defining the key concepts and scope of the book, setting the scene and explaining the rationale. Recognising that there is a wide range of terminology used internationally – and often interchangeably – within the field of practice-based learning, we identify and define the terminology used in this book, ensuring consistency and a shared understanding. This chapter also considers the key stakeholders within allied health practice placement – learners, practice educators and university, college or higher education institutes – and considers what makes a good placement from

DOI: 10.4324/9781003411765-1

these key stakeholder perspectives. Finally, this chapter presents the structure of this book to provide a guide as to how to engage with this 'how-to' toolkit.

CHAPTER OBJECTIVES

The objectives of this chapter are the following.

- Outline the focus, scope and rationale for this book.
- Provide clarity and definition of the terminology that will be adopted within the book and recommended for use within wider practice.
- Consider key stakeholders of practice educators, learners and the university, and outline their expectations of what makes a good placement.
- Outline the content of this chapter and how the book should be used to support adopting new ways of engaging with practice-based learning.

INTRODUCTION: A FOCUS ON THE ALLIED HEALTH PROFESSIONS

This book is designed for practitioners, educators, practice educators and learners with a keen interest in practice-based learning. It is an essential resource for any allied health professional involved in shaping the future workforce and supporting the delivery of effective practice-based learning experiences. Allied health professionals are a diverse group of health and social care workers who play a crucial role in improving the health and wellbeing of populations worldwide, working alongside medicine and nursing. While definitions of which professions fall under allied health vary globally, there is consensus that it includes health and social care professionals who require a university degree and professional registration upon qualifying, excluding the professions of medicine, dentistry and nursing (ASAHP, 2015). Higher education institutes deliver allied health programmes, which are highly regulated by national and international standards to ensure safe, effective and ethical practice (Bissett et al., 2023). This book supports those working in these programmes, offering valuable insights into developing future professionals and fostering excellence in practice-based learning.

Allied health pre-registration programmes typically follow a modular curriculum that integrates academic learning with essential practice-based learning experiences, which are crucial for developing competence to practice (Rodger et al., 2008). However, there is considerable variation across professions regarding the number of required practice hours required, the timing of placements and the diversity of practice settings (Bissett et al., 2023). Accrediting bodies for allied health often outline who can supervise placements, identifying certain models of placements that can be utilised, and for how many hours, e.g., use of simulation. However, often there is no specific guidance on the types and models of placement that can be used (Beveridge and Pentland, 2020). International or national standards within professions may also determine the criteria for this, e.g., the World Federation for Occupational Therapy (WFOT) (2016) requires 1,000 hours practice education for qualification for all WFOT accredited occupational therapy programmes, or criteria can be decided at a national level by professional bodies, e.g., the Royal College of Occupational Therapists (RCOT) sets a limit of 40 hours of simulation only that can be counted within the 1,000 hours required to graduate an occupational therapist (RCOT, 2019). However, although the configuration of the exact criteria may vary from profession to profession and country to country, there is commonality in that allied health profession education includes multiple practice-based learning opportunities designed to develop learners' capabilities and ensure that they meet the required proficiency and work readiness upon graduation (Nagarajan and McAllister, 2015). The flexibility in placement models offers the opportunity for creativity and innovation, allowing educators to tackle global challenges related to placement capacity in allied health (Briffa and Porter, 2013; Pope et al., 2023). This book responds to the shared need for a wide range of practice-based learning opportunities that align with regulatory or professional accreditation standards, whilst also addressing the increasing demand for placement capacity in pre-registration allied health education. In this context, the book provides practical solutions and guidance for universities, practice educators, practitioners and learners. It explores a range of contemporary approaches to practice-based learning, offering strategies to help meet current and future requirements for allied health students and ensure their competence as graduates.

WHAT IS PRACTICE-BASED LEARNING?

Practice-based learning for the allied health professions exists at the junction of academic work and work-based practice, serving as a kind of bridge or transition between university-based, classroom learning and the messy realities of practice (Schön, 1991). The complexity of professional practice has been described by Schön (1991, p. 42) as the "swampy lowlands" where these complex messy situations defy easy technical solutions. This 'betwixt and between' position is both what makes practice-based learning so interesting, but also what can make it so challenging. Compounding this, the terminology surrounding practice-based learning is broad, inconsistent, and varies across professions and countries, with many terms being used interchangeably (Pope et al., 2023). This lack of a unified approach can lead to confusion and a lack of consensus in practice and research (Beveridge and Pentland, 2020). Practice-based learning is an educational approach that emphasises applying theoretical knowledge in real-world practical settings. It serves as an umbrella term for a variety of learning experiences, all designed to foster student-centred learning by providing learners a safe environment to apply and refine their newly acquired knowledge and skills (Chartered Society of Physiotherapy [CSP], 2023). Internationally, the term 'work-integrated learning' is often used synonymously with practice-based learning. In the context of allied health, work-integrated learning has been described as

> *carefully designed learning activities, in a variety of settings, [that] provide allied health students with opportunities to develop abilities to integrate conceptual and procedural knowledge obtained during their on-campus studies with the know-how to make decisions about applying knowledge (such as propositional, procedural, personal, ethical and cultural knowledge) gained.*
>
> (Nagarajan and McAllister, 2015, p. 280)

While these definitions highlight the importance of bridging theoretical knowledge with practical application, they do not capture the full scope of what practice-based learning can offer. Beyond technical skills and knowledge, placement provides crucial experiences in professional socialisation and understanding team dynamics and working relationships, both within professions and across interdisciplinary teams (Rodger et al., 2008). Additionally, it gives learners the opportunity to develop their professional identity and build self-confidence (Snell et al., 2020).

Practice-based learning is typically supported and supervised by qualified practice educators who guide learners' towards achieving specific learning outcomes and assess their competence for practice. This assessment covers both hard competencies, such as technical skills relevant to the profession, and soft competencies, including empathy, values, communication, teamwork and service user–centred approaches (Koh et al., 2022; Rossiter et al., 2023). Practice-based learning can take place in various settings, both on and off campus. On-campus examples include simulation or research placements, though these can also occur in real-world settings. Off-campus experiences might be in a wide range of practice or administrative settings. These practice-based learning experiences are described by different terms across contexts and professions – such as clinical education/experiences, practice, placement, practice learning, fieldwork, work-based learning and practicum – but all refer to opportunities whereby learners engage in practical, hands-on learning. In this book, we use the term 'practice-based learning' intentionally to emphasise the active learning process that occurs in real-world settings, rather than the more passive process of simply being 'placed' somewhere. This aligns with the Allied Health Principles for Practice-Based Learning published in the United Kingdom (UK) (CSP, 2023). The term also encompasses the widely recognised four pillars of practice: education, practice, research and leadership (HEE, 2017). This broad definition reflects the diverse areas within which allied health learners can gain practice-based experience, preparing them for a holistic professional role.

Within practice-based learning there are a range of other terms used interchangeably. The following terminology (Table 1.1) will be used for consistency and clarity of understanding throughout the book.

Table 1.1 Terminology

Preferred term for this book	Definition	Other recognised terms
Practice-based learning	A range of learning experiences (on campus or in practice settings) that facilitate student-centred learning by providing learners a safe environment to apply and practice their newly acquired knowledge and skills (CSP, 2023). It provides learning opportunities to develop professional socialisation, self-confidence and identity within the context of professional practice within uni-professional and interprofessional team working spaces.	Work-based learning, work-integrated learning, fieldwork, placement, practicum, practice education, clinical education, practicum (prac)
Placement	A practice placement is a discrete period of structured and supervised learning whereby learners consolidate and develop learning by applying theoretical knowledge within work placement context to develop competencies for safe, effective, and ethical professional practice.	Practicum, fieldwork, clinical, practicals
Model of placement	A particular learning design approach to developing a placement, normally based on learning theories to facilitate and optimise student learning and support delivery of efficient and effective practice-based learning.	Placement models, placement approaches

Table 1.1 continued

Preferred term for this book	Definition	Other recognised terms
Learners or students	Learner is the student registered on the allied health programme who is engaging in the programme of study. Learners, students and apprentices reflect the growth and development of different routes into the allied health professions – and therefore, simply using the term student no longer encapsulates these developments (CSP, 2023). Therefore, it is becoming widespread practice to adopt the more global and inclusive term of 'learner' as a collective term for a student or apprentice and recognises these different pre-registration routes now available.	Students, apprentices
Practice educator	A practice educator is an appropriately qualified individual who is responsible for facilitating, supervising and assessing learners within placement. Practice educator is also a more inclusive and reflective term of the diverse role beyond just a clinical setting within which practice-based learning can take place (CSP, 2023). Therefore, the term 'practice educator' will be used within this book.	Supervisor, clinical educator, mentor

WHY THIS BOOK?

Traditionally, practice-based learning has been understood as a process whereby learners engage in practical, patient or service user–related activities with the supervision of a qualified professional employed within the service (Rose and Best, 2005). This has often been delivered through an apprenticeship model, whereby one practice educator is assigned to one learner in a clinical or practice setting (Rodger et al., 2008; Beveridge and Pentland, 2020). This model has long dominated practice-based learning in many allied health professions, and it continues to be a widely used approach. However, while this traditional model has proven effective, it does not fully account for advances in our understanding of how students learn, nor does it consider the importance of developing skills beyond patient-facing roles, such as in research and leadership. Additionally, economic, political and societal shifts are putting pressure on the sustainability of the one-to-one apprenticeship model as the primary approach. This book addresses these challenges, offering a practical guide to rethinking and diversifying the delivery of practice-based learning. It explores new models and strategies that are better suited to today's realities, equipping allied health educators, practitioners and learners with tools to expand learning beyond the traditional scope while ensuring students are well prepared for the evolving demands of the healthcare environment.

Health and social care services are currently facing significant workforce demands, which are putting immense pressure on existing finite resources and challenging the sustainability of current practices, including practice-based learning. The global challenge of an increasingly ageing population – who are living longer but often with higher levels of frailty and comorbidities – exacerbates this issue. Coupled with medical advances which mean that children and adults are living longer, with higher levels of disability, and with a complex context of social justice issues affecting people's health and wellbeing is challenging health and social care services and practice-based learning. In response to these challenges, strategies are emerging that advocate for an early intervention and preventive approach to service delivery, emphasising collaboration with groups, communities, and society at large, rather than a focus on one-on-one interactions. This evolving landscape of need, alongside broader societal changes, necessitates a modernisation of practice-based learning. It is essential to equip learners with the skills to work collaboratively and effectively in teams across various settings, preparing future allied health professionals for the realities they will face in their careers (Markowski et al., 2021). Moreover, the current climate in health and social care has intensified the challenges related to workforce capacity among allied health professionals, directly affecting placement availability. This situation highlights the urgent need to explore alternative models of placement to ensure that future professionals receive the education and experience necessary to thrive in their roles (Pope et al., 2023)

A central rationale for this book is the recognition of the need to modernise the approach to practice-based learning. It introduces a variety of placement models and learning approaches that offer meaningful alternatives to the traditional one-to-one apprenticeship style. The models and examples presented in this book emphasise peer learning as a key element, shifting the role of the practice educator from the director of learning to a facilitator of learning opportunities. This reflects advances in our understanding of how adults learn within social and real-world contexts (Bandura and Walters, 1977; Lave and Wenger, 1991). alongside the more recent conceptualisation of the "professional development crucible" that outlines work-related learning as a situational, relational, and temporal experience (Patton et al., 2018, p. 135). This model provides an articulation of the complexity of practice-based learning by identifying four key spaces that are fluid and interact to develop students professional practice capabilities: workplace influences, clinical supervisors' intentions and actions, students' disposition and experiences and engagement in professional practices (Patton et al., 2018). By incorporating peer learning and recognition of spaces within the "professional development crucible" (Patton et al., 2018, p. 136), these models of placement encourage collaboration among learners and educators noting these contextual, relational and social elements of learning, fostering engagement with all four pillars of practice: clinical practice, education, research and leadership (HEE, 2017). This broader approach moves beyond the traditional focus on developing only practice skills and competencies, highlighting the importance of cultivating a well-rounded professional capable of thriving in various aspects of allied health.

WHO IS THIS BOOK FOR, AND WHAT ARE THEIR EXPECTATIONS OF A "GOOD" PLACEMENT?

This book has been written for anyone with an interest in practice-based learning, including learners, universities and practice educators. In line with the UK allied health "Principles of Practice-Based Learning" (CSP, 2023), it aims to demystify the practical aspects of designing and implementing various placement models by drawing on both evidence-based research and real-world examples. The goal is to support all stakeholders by providing a clear understanding of different placement models and offering practical guidance on their effective design and implementation. However, each stakeholder – whether students, practice educators or universities or higher education institutions – has unique expectations, needs and priorities when it comes to practice-based learning. These differing perspectives shape how placement models are applied in practice. Therefore, it is essential to consider general good practice principles for each stakeholder group when engaging with this book, ensuring placements are effective and beneficial for everyone involved.

A 'good' placement: learners' perspective

From a learner's perspective, a 'good' allied health placement is one whereby they feel connected, supported and valued, providing a safe and inclusive learning environment for developing clinical and professional skills. Majeed (2017) emphasises that positive placements are those which students speak about favourably, with a manageable workload that balances hands-on experience with time for reflection. Supportive supervisors who offer guidance appropriate to the student's level are crucial for creating meaningful learning experiences. Conversely, placements lacking these elements can lead to stress, demoralisation and even burnout for both learners and staff.

A keen sense of belonging and psychological safety is essential for student engagement, allowing them to learn confidently without fear of judgement or feeling like a burden (Brentnall et al., 2024). This can be fostered through small yet impactful actions, such as learning students' names and pronunciations, providing a clear induction and structured timetable (particularly in early weeks of placement), ensuring team inclusion, clarifying workplace norms (e.g., lunch breaks) and accommodating cultural and religious considerations. Constructive feedback is also crucial for helping students refine their skills and knowledge while ensuring fair assessment based on their learning stage (Judd et al., 2023). Students appreciate recognition for their progress and benefit from linking theoretical knowledge to practical applications, ensuring that they are succeeding in placement learning for future practice (Judd et al., 2023).

Adequate preparation in both practical and theoretical aspects is vital, as feeling unprepared can hinder student confidence (Davenport et al., 2018). Supervision should strike a balance between guidance and independence, allowing students to build their confidence while ensuring patient safety (Dancza et al., 2023). When these factors are in place, students are more likely to have a positive placement experience, develop professional competence and transition effectively into their roles as allied health professionals.

A 'good' placement: practice educators' perspective

From a practice educator's perspective, a 'good' allied health placement provides a structured yet flexible learning environment whereby students can develop clinical skills, critical thinking and professional behaviours. Clear communication and well-defined expectations between students, educators and the broader healthcare team are essential for ensuring a productive placement experience (Health and Care Professions Council, 2020). Practice educators value placements whereby students are well-prepared, professional and proactive in their learning, demonstrating a willingness to engage with feedback and reflect on their practice (Boud and Molloy, 2013). This is often built from a 'good' relationship with the learner (Evans et al., 2024). Effective supervision, balancing support with independence, allows students to build confidence and competence while ensuring patient safety. The 3 Cs model – connections, content and continuing development – is recommended as an effective supervision framework (Dancza et al., 2023).

Adaptability is also crucial for practice educators; while structured learning opportunities are important, the ability to respond to unexpected challenges fosters resilience and problem-solving skills in students and practice educators to support learning (Evans et al., 2024). Practice educators also value placements that incorporate evidence-based practice and provide real-world examples to help students link theory to practice (Hoffman et al., 2017). Practice educators often see their role primarily as assessors rather than educators, expecting students to meet competency requirements and ensuring fair, constructive evaluations of their progress (Norcini et al., 2018). To ensure that placements are effective for both students and practice educators, continuous evaluation and reflection are essential. This process should be ongoing, not limited to the end of the placement, to promote continuous improvement and a supportive learning environment. Regular feedback allows for timely adjustments, ensuring placements remain responsive and aligned with students' learning objectives and individual needs (Penman et al., 2021).

A 'good' placement: university/higher education perspective

From a university's perspective, high-quality allied health placements are crucial for student progression to support graduates enter the workforce. Universities expect practice educator to provide clear action plans addressing learning needs and explicit, ongoing feedback with actionable steps for improvement. They value strong partnerships between universities and placement providers, whereby communication and collaboration ensure that students receive consistent, supportive learning experiences (Health and Care Professions Council, 2020). A good placement offers a range of learning opportunities that allow students to demonstrate competencies while developing their employability and professional identity (Boud and Molloy, 2013). Universities also emphasise the importance of linking learning theories to real-world practice, helping students make meaningful connections between academic knowledge and its application in clinical settings (Yardley et al., 2012). Reflection time is prioritised, ensuring that students have time to consolidate their experiences without being overwhelmed by excessive scheduling. A flexible approach to evidencing learning outcomes is also important, enabling students to demonstrate their progress in a way that aligns with their unique learning preferences and experience and diverse needs (Patton et al., 2018). Universities seek placements that foster professional development in a safe and supported learning environment, enabling students to grow both clinically and professionally in preparation for their future careers.

HOW TO USE THIS BOOK

This book is designed to support practice educators, universities and learners in understanding, implementing and engaging with various models of placement. It caters to a broad audience, including university and college lecturers interested in practice-based learning, learners who have been allocated specific types of placements and wish to understand their implications, and practice educators looking to explore or enhance their understanding and application of contemporary approaches to practice-based learning. With a strong emphasis on educational design, this book serves as a practical guide for educators and practice educators, particularly those new to innovative placement models. Recognising the critical role that practice educators play in planning, designing, supporting, delivering, and assessing practice-based learning experiences – whether in clinical, research or leadership contexts – this book is specifically crafted to equip them with the knowledge and tools necessary to enrich the learning experiences of future allied health professionals.

The first two chapters provide essential context for practice-based learning within allied health professions. Chapter 2 summarises the existing challenges and opportunities within the health and social care landscape, outlining future workforce needs and demands through the lens of practice-based learning. Chapter 3 introduces concepts of equity, diversity and belonging from a practice-based learning perspective, highlighting current challenges faced by allied health learners and offering strategies to address these issues moving forward. These two chapters provide the reader with an overview of the general issues and practice strategies for considering how we support the future development of allied health professionals in an inclusive way.

The following nine chapters present a variety of approaches to practice-based learning. Some of these relate to educational approaches, such as peer-assisted learning considering same-level and near-peer approaches (Chapter 4), others the approach to supervision, such as long-arm supervision (Chapter 6), and the modes of delivery of placement, e.g., technology-enabled placements: online, virtual and hybrid (Chapter 6). The final six chapters provide detailed 'how-to' guidance for a range of models of placement available to support practice-based learning for allied health learners. Readers are encouraged to 'pick and mix' chapters that are relevant to their specific interests, combining them to design and develop innovative approaches to practice-based learning. Notably, Chapters 7–12, which outline different placement models, emphasise that optimal delivery should incorporate peer-assisted learning. Therefore, it is recommended that these chapters be read in conjunction with Chapter 4 to maximise their effectiveness.

REFERENCES

Association of Schools Advancing Health Professions. (2015). *Definition of allied health*. Available at: What is allied health? – ASAHP. (Accessed 24 March 2025).

Bandura, A. and Walters, R. H. (1977). *Social Learning Theory* (Vol. 1). Englewood Cliffs, NJ: Prentice Hall.

Beveridge, J. and Pentland, D. (2020). A mapping review of models of practice education in allied health and social care professions. *British Journal of Occupational Therapy*, *83*(8), pp. 488–513.

Bissett, M., Tuttle, N. and Cardell, E. (2023). Allied health education: Current and future trends. In D. Nestle, G. Reedy, L. McKenna and S. Gough (Eds.), *Clinical Education for the Health Professions: Theory and Practice* (pp. 135–151). Springer.

Boud, D. and Molloy, E. (2013). *Feedback in Higher and Professional Education: Understanding It and Doing It Well*. Routledge.

Brentnall, J., Rossiter, L., Judd, B., et al. (2024). Education design insights for interprofessional immersive simulation to prepare allied health students for clinical placements. *Advances in Simulation*, *9*(45). https://doi.org/10.1186/s41077-024-00316-0

Briffa, C. and Porter, J. (2013). A systematic review of the collaborative clinical education model to inform speech-language pathology practice. *International Journal of Speech-Language Pathology*, *15*(6), pp. 564–574.

Chartered Society of Physiotherapy. (2023). *AHP principles of practice-based learning*. CSP London. Available at: https://www.csp.org.uk/system/files/publication_files/AHP%20Principles%20of%20Practice-based%20Learning_Digital_Oct23_Final.pdf (Accessed 1 March 2024).

Dancza, K., Volkert, A. and Tempest, S. (2023). *Supervision for Occupational Therapy: Practical Guidance for Supervisors and Supervisees*. Abingdon, Oxon: Routledge.

Davenport, R., Hewat, S., Ferguson, A., McAllister, S. and Lincoln, M. (2018). Struggle and failure on clinical placement: A critical narrative review. *International Journal of Language & Communication Disorders*, *53*(2), pp. 218–227.

Evans, G., Penman, M. and Thomson, K. (2024). Clinical educator expertise: A scoping review. *The Clinical Teacher*, *21*(4). https://doi.org/10.1111/tct.13729

Health and Care Professions Council. (2020). *Standards of Conduct, Performance, and Ethics*. London: Health and Care Professions Council.

Higher Education England. (2017). *Multi-professional framework for advanced clinical practice in England*. Available at: https://www.hee.nhs.uk/sites/default/files/documents/multi-professionalframeworkforadvancedclinicalpracticeinengland.pdf (Accessed 24 March 2025).

Hoffman, T., Bennett, S. and Del Mar, C. (2017). *Evidence-Based Practice Across the Health Professions*. Elsevier.

Judd, B., Brentnall, J., Scanlan, J. N., et al. (2023). Evaluating allied health students' readiness for placement learning. *BMC Medical Education*, 23(70). https://doi.org/10.1186/s12909-023-04005-w

Koh, J. M. Y., Ang, H. G., Lee, J. and Pua, Y. H. (2022). The hard truth about soft skills: Exploring the association between leadership competency and career advancement of allied health professionals. *Proceedings of Singapore Healthcare*, *31*, p. 20101058221138834.

Lave, J. and Wenger, E. (1991). *Situated Learning: Legitimate Peripheral Participation*. Cambridge, UK: Cambridge University Press.

Majeed, A. (2017). *What makes a good clinical training placement?* Imperial Medical Centre Blogs. Available at: What makes a good clinical training placement? – Medical Centre. (Accessed 18 December 2024).

Markowski, M., Bower, H., Essex, R. and Yearley, C. (2021). Peer learning and collaborative placement models in health care: A systematic review and qualitative synthesis of the literature. *Journal of Clinical Nursing*, *30*(11–12), pp. 1519–1541.

Nagarajan, S. V. and McAllister, L. (2015). Integration of practice experiences into the allied health curriculum: Curriculum and pedagogic considerations before, during and after work-integrated learning experiences. *Asia-Pacific Journal of Cooperative Education*, *16*(4), pp. 279–290.

Norcini, J., Anderson, M. B., Bollela, V., Burch, V., Joao Costa, M., Duvivier, R., Hays, R., Mackay, M. F. P., Roberts, T. and Swanson, D. (2018). 2108 Consensus framework for good assessment. *Medical Teacher*, *40*(11), pp. 1102–1109. https://doi.org/10.1080/0142159X.2018.1500016

Patton, N., Higgs, J. and Smith, M. (Eds.). (2018). *Developing Practice Capability: Transforming Workplace Learning*. Boston: BRILL. Available at: ProQuest ebook central. (Accessed 22 March 2025).

Penman, M., Tai, J., Thompson, T. and Thomson, K. (2021). Feedback practices as part of signature pedagogy for clinical placements. *Assessment in Education: Principles, Policy & Practice*, *28*(2), pp. 151–169. https://doi.org/10.1080/0969594X.2021.1892587

Pope, K., Barclay, L., Dixon, K. and Kent, F. (2023). Models of pre-registration student supervision in allied health: A scoping review. *Focus on Health Professional Education: A Multi-Professional Journal*, *24*(2), pp. 27–62.

Rodger, S., Thomas, Y., Fitzgerald, C., Dickson, D., McBryde, C., Edwards, A., Broadbridge, J. and Hawkins, R. (2008). Evaluation of a collaborative project to engage occupational therapy clinicians in promoting practice placement education. *British Journal of Occupational Therapy*, *71*(6), pp. 248–252.

Rose, M. L. and Best, D. L. (Eds.). (2005). *Transforming Practice through Clinical Education, Professional Supervision, and Mentoring*. Elsevier Health Sciences.

Rossiter, L., Turk, R., Judd, B., Brentnall, J., Grimmett, C., Cowley, E., McCormick, K. and Thackray, D. (2023). Preparing allied health students for placement: A contrast of learning modalities for foundational skill development. *BMC Medical Education*, *23*(1), p. 161.

Royal College of Occupational Therapists. (2019). *Learning and Development Standards for Pre-Registration Education*. London: Royal College of Occupational Therapists.

Schön, D. A. (1991). *The Reflective Practitioner: How Professionals Think in Action*. Ashgate Publishing.

Snell, R., Fyfe, S., Fyfe, G., Blackwood, D. and Itsiopoulos, C. (2020). Development of professional identity and professional socialisation in allied health students: A scoping review. *Focus on Health Professional Education: A Multi-Professional Journal*, *21*(1), p. 29.

World Federation for Occupational Therapy. (2016). *Minimum Standards for the Education of Occupational Therapists*. World Federation of Occupational Therapists.

Yardley, S., Teunissen, P. W. and Dornan, T. (2012). Experiential learning: Transforming theory into practice. *Medical Teacher*, *34*(2), pp. e102–e108.

Chapter 2

Future workforce and practice

Individuals, groups, communities and populations

Anita Volkert, Kerryn Dillon and Lisa Forrest

CHAPTER OVERVIEW

The future landscape of health and social care demands a nuanced understanding of emerging trends, challenges and strategies to effectively navigate workforce dynamics, and this understanding is crucial to the planning and provision of practice education across the allied health professions. This chapter provides a comprehensive exploration of the evolving nature of the health and social care workforce, offering insights into the transformative forces shaping its trajectory which in turn influence student placement learning. Key topics include the impact of technological advancements, demographic shifts and evolving healthcare delivery models on workforce composition and the skills requirements of students as evolving practitioners. Furthermore, the chapter delves into the complexities of workforce recruitment, retention and training amidst growing demand and resource constraints. Drawing on interdisciplinary perspectives, it examines innovative approaches to workforce development, including the integration of digital health technologies, interprofessional collaboration and community-based care initiatives. By critically analysing current practices and envisioning future possibilities, this chapter aims to inform policymakers, educators and practitioners about the evolving landscape of health and social care workforce, and to equip them with actionable strategies to address the challenges and seize the opportunities of tomorrow.

DOI: 10.4324/9781003411765-2

CHAPTER OBJECTIVES

The objectives of this chapter are the following.

- To provide a critical analysis of the practice and education context of the allied health professions, currently and in the future.
- To discuss some of the solutions to the identified societal, political, educational and workplace challenges as they pertain to student practice learning.

INTRODUCTION

The health and social care sector faces an evolving array of challenges and opportunities. As the global population ages and the burden of chronic diseases increases, the demand for a skilled and adaptable health workforce becomes more pressing. Integral to the development of this workforce is the experience gained through placements and fieldwork. This chapter explores the critical link between these hands-on learning experiences and the preparation of future healthcare professionals, examining how placements and fieldwork influence competency, confidence and career trajectories.

THE ROLE OF PLACEMENTS AND FIELDWORK IN HEALTH AND SOCIAL CARE EDUCATION

Placements and fieldwork are structured educational experiences that occur in real-world settings. These experiences are essential components of health education programmes, offering students the opportunity to apply theoretical knowledge, develop practical skills and understand the dynamics of healthcare delivery. The immersive nature of placements allows students to achieve the following.

Integrate theory and practice: Students can see the direct application of their classroom learning in practice settings, reinforcing their understanding and enabling them to bridge the gap between theory and practice.

Develop clinical skills: Hands-on practice is crucial for mastering clinical procedures, diagnostic techniques and service user–interaction skills. Fieldwork provides a supervised environment where students can hone these abilities.

Build professional competence: Exposure to real-world scenarios helps students develop critical thinking, problem solving and decision-making skills. It also fosters adaptability and resilience, essential traits for health and social care professionals.

Gain insights into healthcare systems: Placements expose students to the complexities of health and social care delivery, including the interdisciplinary nature of care, the importance of communication and the impact of organisational structures on patient and service-user outcomes.

Enhancing competency through fieldwork

Competency in healthcare is multifaceted, encompassing clinical proficiency, ethical practice and the ability to work within a team. Fieldwork experiences play a pivotal role in enhancing the following competencies.

Clinical proficiency: Repeated exposure to clinical settings allows students to refine their technical skills. Regular feedback from supervisors and mentors is crucial in this learning process, helping students to correct errors and improve their techniques.

Ethical and professional practice: Real-world experiences challenge students to navigate ethical dilemmas and professional boundaries. This exposure is essential for developing a strong ethical foundation and understanding the importance of professional conduct.

Team collaboration: Health and social professionals work in multidisciplinary teams. Fieldwork provides opportunities for students to collaborate with various healthcare providers, understand distinct roles and appreciate the importance of teamwork in service-user care.

Confidence building through practical experience

Confidence is a critical attribute for healthcare professionals, affecting their performance and patient interactions. Placements and fieldwork are instrumental in building this confidence.

Experiential learning: Direct service-user care experiences help students gain confidence in their abilities. As they become more familiar with clinical environments and procedures, their self-assurance grows.

Mentorship and support: Positive relationships with mentors and supervisors during placements can significantly boost students' confidence. Constructive feedback and encouragement help students feel more competent and prepared for professional practice.

Overcoming challenges: Fieldwork often presents unexpected challenges and complex cases. Successfully navigating these situations enhances students' confidence in their problem-solving and critical thinking skills.

Career development and workforce preparedness

Placements and fieldwork are also crucial for career development and readiness to enter the workforce.

Networking opportunities: During placements, students have the chance to build professional networks. These connections can lead to job opportunities, references and mentorship beyond their educational programmes.

Career clarification: Exposure to different specialties and settings helps students clarify their career interests and goals. Fieldwork can illuminate paths they might not have considered and confirm their passion for specific areas of healthcare.

Job market readiness: Employers look for candidates with practical experience. Fieldwork provides the hands-on experience required for students to qualify in their chosen field and show evidence of their transferable skills gained through practice education.

Challenges and opportunities in placements and fieldwork

While the benefits of placements and fieldwork are clear, there are also challenges and opportunities for improvement.

Access and availability: Ensuring that all students have access to quality placements can be difficult, particularly in underserved areas. Innovative solutions, such as telehealth placements or partnerships with a broader range of healthcare providers, can help address these gaps.

Standardisation and quality: Variability in placement experiences can affect the consistency of learning outcomes. Establishing clear standards and guidelines for placements can help ensure that all students receive high-quality training.

Support systems: Students often face stress and burnout during placements. Providing robust support systems, including mental health resources and peer support networks, is essential for maintaining their wellbeing.

THE FUTURE HEALTH AND SOCIAL CARE WORKFORCE

The future of healthcare provision is rapidly evolving, driven by a myriad of complex factors such as technological advancements, demographic shifts and changing health and social care needs, such as responding to predicted future crises, preparing for increased use of digital technologies and planning for demographic change (Cometto et al., 2020; International Labour Organization, 2022; Codd et al., 2023). Looking ahead, it is essential when preparing for and implementing practice-based learning to consider the future health workforce and how it will adapt to meet the growing demands and complexities of health and social care delivery (Cometto et al., 2020; Fleming, 2023; Carmona and Trujillo, 2023). This chapter delves into the various facets of the future health workforce, including challenges, opportunities and the role of emerging technologies. It explores the need for a more diverse and skilled health workforce, the impact of telemedicine and artificial intelligence (AI), and the importance of workforce planning to ensure a sustainable healthcare system. We also touch upon global perspectives to provide a well-rounded view of this critical issue to the understanding and implementation of student practice–based learning (Balasubramanian and Short, 2021).

WHAT DOES THE EVIDENCE TELL US?

The health and social care landscape is undergoing a transformation driven by a range of factors, including advances in technology, shifting demographics and changing patient expectations. The traditional model of healthcare, with its emphasis on in-person visits to healthcare facilities, is giving way to a more service user–centric, technology-enabled and efficient system (Cometto et al., 2020; Maeda and Socha-Dietrich, 2021), although one that may work with much more geo-political and social unpredictability in terms of epidemiology, climate and disaster (Okoroafor et al., 2022). As we stand on the cusp of this healthcare evolution, one of the critical considerations is the future of the health and social care workforce and, crucially, how we prepare that workforce through student practice education (Fleming, 2023).

The health and social care workforce comprise a diverse group of professionals, including physicians, nurses, allied health practitioners, technicians, support workers delivering direct care, and administrative staff. These individuals form the backbone of the healthcare system, providing clinical care, support, and administrative services (Karan et al., 2021). The effectiveness, quality and accessibility of healthcare services depend heavily on the composition and capabilities of the health and social care workforce (Cometto et al., 2020). Leerapan et al. (2021) found that a focus on hospital care in health and social care policy planning created a vicious cycle of constantly increasing demands for this care and a constant shortage of healthcare providers. They argue that such care is not designed to effectively dealing with the future demands of ageing populations and prevalent chronic illness. Hence, shifting the emphasis to professions that can provide primary, intermediate, long-term, palliative and end-of-life care can be much more effective (Leerapan et al., 2021). This shift may include a larger emphasis on the allied health professions (Anderson et al., 2021; Leerapan et al., 2021), and hence a larger focus in the education and practice learning experiences of student allied health professionals.

Indeed, one of the most significant challenges facing the future health workforce is the ageing population. Both the Global North and South are experiencing a demographic shift with the ageing of the older generation, often referred to in the Global North as the baby boomer generation (Cheng et al., 2020). As this large cohort continues to age, there is and will continue to be a surge in demand for healthcare services, particularly for chronic disease management and geriatric care (Han et al., 2020). This places immense pressure on health and social care systems to provide adequate staffing and resources to meet these needs (Cometto et al., 2020). Conversely, the workforce itself is changing. A younger generation of Millennials and Generation Z are entering the healthcare field with different expectations and work preferences. They are usually tech-savvy, value work–life balance and seek opportunities for career advancement. Adapting healthcare workplaces to accommodate these generational differences and retaining talent will be crucial (Locke et al., 2022; Hardin, 2020). Furthermore, the increasing pressure of the work and generational differences between educators and students in the practice context provide a well-documented challenge to overcome.

Health disparities, often rooted in injustices within the social determinants of health, continue to persist in many parts of the world, in both the Global North and South (Hickson, 2024). These disparities are complex and rooted in history, and they affect every aspect of human body function, structure, activity and participation (Eadie, 2003). In addition, these disparities are reflected in the composition of the health workforce itself. Addressing health inequities requires a diverse and culturally competent workforce that can understand and cater to the unique needs of various communities. Achieving this diversity remains a challenge, especially in areas with historical underrepresentation (Myers and Dreachslin, 2007; Pittman et al., 2021). As health and social care students become more diverse to reflect the populations they serve, their historically less diverse educators may struggle to implement contemporary approaches to practice education which are required to engage a more diverse population of students and adequately facilitate their learning.

Workforce shortages in various healthcare professions are a pressing issue. Both medical and allied health professionals are in high demand, and shortages can lead to delayed access to care and increased healthcare costs (Agyeman-Manu et al.,

2023). Rural areas are particularly vulnerable to these shortages, as they struggle to attract and retain healthcare providers (Fahs and Rouhana, 2020). Additionally, many countries experience problems with qualified health and social care professionals and workers dropping out of the labour market and not returning, or having too many unqualified versus qualified workers (Karan et al., 2021). As practice educators are drawn from the existing workforce, these shortages can create a bottleneck of ever larger student cohorts, with ever smaller professional workforces with which to provide practice education.

Healthcare professionals in practice also face increasingly elevated levels of stress and burnout due to heavy workloads, long hours and the emotional toll of caring for patients, especially during and after the COVID-19 pandemic (Leo et al., 2021). The mental health and wellbeing of the workforce are critical concerns that need to be addressed to ensure a sustainable and resilient healthcare system (Maeda and Socha-Dietrich, 2021). With population emotional health and wellbeing at an all-time low (Butterworth et al., 2020), particularly amongst the young people who make up a substantial proportion of student health and social care professionals, the mental health, wellbeing and resilience of the future workforce needs to be considered at student level as well as at workforce level.

FUTURE HEALTH WORKFORCE: OPPORTUNITIES

Telemedicine and telehealth have emerged as powerful tools for expanding access to healthcare services. The ability to provide care remotely can help bridge geographical gaps and improve healthcare access in underserved areas. Telehealth also offers opportunities for asynchronous care, enabling providers to reach more patients while optimising their schedules (Blandford et al., 2020), and provides opportunities for students to be supervised remotely, enabling them to both take on responsibility with the safety net of constant supervision if required, or to undertake placement experiences with rural and remote communities with support. It is important that students have experiences of telehealth during their education, and if possible, during placement experiences, as early exposure to these approaches has been shown to be beneficial to a range of learning outcomes, such as situational awareness, collaborative practice, and decision-making.

AI and machine learning (ML) are revolutionising healthcare in several ways. These technologies can assist in diagnosis, predict disease outbreaks and streamline administrative tasks. AI-powered chatbots and virtual assistants can handle routine patient inquiries, freeing up healthcare professionals for more complex tasks (Alowais et al., 2023; Sarker, 2024). Again, these have applicability to the student population, providing answers to questions if a supervisor is unavailable, orienting students to the theory that underpins their practice decision-making and providing them with quick access to the evidence that they may need to make a practice decision.

The future health workforce will need to embrace interdisciplinary collaboration much more than is currently the norm to provide holistic service-user care (Ross, 2024). This includes breaking down silos between healthcare professions and encouraging teamwork among physicians, nurses, pharmacists, social workers and all other allied health professionals (Maeda and Socha-Dietrich, 2021). Collaborative care models can lead to better service-user outcomes and more efficient resource utilisation, particularly when the service user(s) are considered part of the collaborative approach (Hughes et al., 2020). It is standard practice for allied health education programmes to include interprofessional approaches to learning, and whilst these approaches may happen naturally on placement as students immerse themselves in interprofessional teams, there is also a place for the deliberate planning of interprofessional student experiences on practice-based learning, and this has been less utilised as a learning approach to date.

A diverse and inclusive workforce is essential for addressing health disparities and providing culturally competent care. Healthcare organisations must actively promote diversity in their hiring practices and create inclusive environments where all employees feel valued and heard. A diverse workforce can better understand and serve the needs of diverse patient populations (Stanford, 2020), but a diverse student population without a matching diverse workforce may provide challenges in the implementation of pedagogical approaches to support truly inclusive, equitable, practice-based learning with an emphasis on welcoming and belonging.

The evolving healthcare landscape is creating opportunities for new roles and specialisations within the health workforce (Crowell and Boynton, 2020). For example, health informaticians are needed to manage and analyse vast amounts of healthcare data, while genetic counsellors are in demand as personalised medicine becomes more prevalent. Adaptable educational programmes – including innovation in placement provision such as practice-based learning opportunities in new and innovative areas – are required to train professionals for these emerging roles (Frenk et al., 2022).

THE ROLE OF EMERGING TECHNOLOGIES

Telemedicine has the potential to revolutionise healthcare access, particularly in rural and underserved areas. Remote consultations can provide medical expertise where it is needed most, reducing the burden of travel for service users, and improving overall health outcomes (Blandford et al., 2020).

Connected devices and wearable technology can enable real-time monitoring of service users with chronic conditions. This not only enhances service-user engagement but also allows healthcare providers to intervene promptly when issues arise, reducing hospital readmissions and accident and emergency visits (Tariq, 2024).

AI algorithms can analyse medical images, such as X-ray and magnetic resonance imaging (MRI) scans, with high accuracy, assisting radiologists in diagnosing diseases like cancer. Additionally, AI-driven treatment recommendations can personalise care plans based on a service user's unique medical history and genetics (Khan and Alotaibi, 2020).

AI-driven analytics can sift through vast datasets to identify patterns and trends, which can inform public health initiatives and improve preventive care strategies. Predictive analytics can help identify high-risk patients and intervene proactively to prevent health crises (Kumar et al., 2023). Robotic surgery systems are increasingly used in procedures, allowing for greater precision and smaller incisions. Automation can also be applied to routine tasks in healthcare facilities, such as medication dispensing and sterilisation processes (Sarker et al., 2021). Administrative tasks, such as appointment scheduling and billing, can be automated through AI-driven chatbots and software. This streamlines administrative processes, reduces errors and frees up healthcare professionals to focus on increasingly complex service-user care (Holland et al., 2021). You can read more about using technology in student education in Chapter 7.

WORKFORCE PLANNING AND EDUCATION

Effective workforce planning involves predicting future healthcare needs based on demographic trends, epidemiology and technological advancements. Governments, healthcare organisations and educational institutions must collaborate to align student numbers, education programme content and workforce development with evolving healthcare demands (Anderson et al., 2021; Balasubramanian and Short, 2021; Cometto et al., 2020).

Educational programmes must adapt to equip future healthcare professionals with the skills and knowledge needed to navigate a technology-driven healthcare landscape. This includes incorporating digital literacy, data analytics, and telemedicine training into curricula. Maeda and Socha-Dietrich (2021) suggest a focus on person-centred communication, interprofessional teamwork, self-awareness and sociocultural sensitivity in pre-registration health and social care courses, and that this focus be carried into practice-based learning environments. This is often described as a focus on 'soft skills' rather than the 'hard skills' of specific clinical competencies.

Continuous learning and upskilling will be essential for health and social care professionals to stay current in their fields and successfully make the shift to values-based care. Online courses, certifications and on-the-job training can help health and social care workers adapt to modern technologies and values-based practices (Vesty et al., 2024). Maeda and Socha-Dietrich (2021) point out the need for health and social care professionals to upskill in areas of communication, teamwork, self-awareness and sociocultural sensitivity, a view supported by Vesty et al. (2024). This is vital as educational programmes for student allied health programmes make this shift; otherwise, the mismatch between the skill sets of students and the workforce risks becoming too great.

Governments play a pivotal role in shaping the future health workforce through policies, funding and incentives for potential students, students and workforce. These can include such measures as scholarship and bursary programmes, loan forgiveness for healthcare professionals serving in underserved areas and regulations that promote telehealth adoption (Anderson et al., 2021).

THE FUTURE HEALTH AND SOCIAL CARE WORKFORCE: A GLOBAL PERSPECTIVE

Healthcare workforce challenges and opportunities are not unique to any country or region. Many countries are grappling with similar issues, such as ageing populations and workforce shortages. International collaboration and knowledge sharing can lead to innovative solutions at the practice-based learning level across the world (Cometto et al., 2020).

Different healthcare systems around the world have adopted a range of successful approaches to both future workforce planning and healthcare delivery. Examining these systems can provide valuable insights into what works and what does not, informing policy decisions locally (International Labour Organization, 2022).

Global collaboration in healthcare research, education and workforce development can accelerate progress in addressing familiar challenges. International partnerships can facilitate the exchange of best practices and promote innovation in both education and healthcare delivery (International Labour Organization, 2022)

CONCLUSION

Placements and fieldwork are indispensable in shaping the future health workforce. They provide essential experiences that enhance competency, build confidence and prepare students for their careers. By addressing the challenges and maximising the opportunities associated with these experiences, educational institutions and healthcare organisations can ensure that the next generation of healthcare professionals is well-equipped to meet the demands of an ever-changing healthcare landscape.

The future health workforce faces a myriad of challenges, including demographic shifts, health inequities, workforce shortages and burnout. Addressing these challenges requires strategic planning, investment and a commitment to promoting diversity and wellbeing within the workforce, as well as attention paid to green issues (Codd et al., 2023).

The integration of emerging technologies such as telemedicine, AI, and automation presents unprecedented opportunities to improve healthcare access, quality and efficiency. Embracing these innovations requires a flexible and forward-thinking health workforce (Nazeha et al., 2020).

The future of healthcare is marked by uncertainty, but also by immense potential. The health workforce of tomorrow must be adaptable, technologically proficient and committed to providing patient-centred care. It is through thoughtful planning and collaboration that we can build, through our students of today, a future health workforce capable of meeting the evolving healthcare needs of society (International Labour Organization, 2022).

REFERENCES

Agyeman-Manu, K., Ghebreyesus, T.A., Maait, M., Rafila, A., Tom, L., Lima, N.T. and Wangmo, D. (2023). Prioritising the health and care workforce shortage: Protect, invest, together. *The Lancet Global Health*, *11*(8), pp. e1162–e1164. https://doi.org/10.1016/S2214-109X(23)00224-3. Epub 2023 May 17. PMID: 37209702; PMCID: PMC10191605.

Alowais, S. A., Alghamdi, S. S., Alsuhebany, N., Alqahtani, T., Alshaya, A. I., Almohareb, S. N., Aldairem, A., Alrashed, M., Bin Saleh, K., Badreldin, H. A. and Al Yami, M. S. (2023). Revolutionizing healthcare: The role of artificial intelligence in clinical practice. *BMC Medical Education*, *23*(1), p. 689.

Anderson, M., O'Neill, C., Clark, J. M., Street, A., Woods, M., Johnston-Webber, C., Charlesworth, A., Whyte, M., Foster, M., Majeed, A. and Pitchforth, E. (2021). Securing a sustainable and fit-for-purpose UK health and care workforce. *The Lancet*, *397*(10288), pp. 1992–2011.

Balasubramanian, M. and Short, S. (2021). The future health workforce: Integrated solutions and models of care. *International Journal of Environmental Research and Public Health*, 18, p. 2849.

Blandford, A., Wesson, J., Amalberti, R., AlHazme, R. and Allwihan, R. (2020). Opportunities and challenges for telehealth within, and beyond, a pandemic. *The Lancet Global Health*, *8*(11), pp. e1364–e1365.

Butterworth, P., Watson, N. and Wooden, M. (2020). Trends in the prevalence of psychological distress over time: Comparing results from longitudinal and repeated cross-sectional surveys. *Frontiers in Psychiatry*, *11*, p. 595696.

Carmona, N. and Trujillo, M. (2023). Developing vaccine literacy for urban health science students, the future health workforce. *Journal of Microbiology & Biology Education*, *24*(2), p. e00038–23.

Cheng, X., Yang, Y., Schwebel, D. C., Liu, Z., Li, L., Cheng, P., Ning, P. and Hu, G. (2020). Population ageing and mortality during 1990–2017: A global decomposition analysis. *PLoS Medicine*, *17*(6), p. e1003138.

Codd, M., Valiotis, G., Davidovitch, N., Kostoulas, P., Razum, O., Mabhala, M., Leighton, L., Otok, R. and Signorelli, C. (2023). Building the future one health workforce. *Eurohealth*, *29*(2), p. 2.

Cometto, G., Buchan, J. and Dussault, G. (2020). Developing the health workforce for universal health coverage. *Bulletin of the World Health Organization*, *98*(2), p. 109.

Crowell, D. M. and Boynton, B. (2020). *Complexity Leadership: Nursing's Role in Health Care Delivery*. FA Davis.

Eadie, T. L. (2003). The ICF: A proposed framework for comprehensive rehabilitation of individuals who use alaryngeal speech. *American Journal of Speech-Language Pathology*, *12*(2), pp. 189–197.

Fahs, P. S. and Rouhana, N. (2020). Rural health care: Workforce challenges and opportunities. *Policy and Politics in Nursing and Health Care*, pp. 437–446.

Fleming, P. (2023). How 2008 financial crisis legacies impacted future health workforce resilience – a realist review. *European Journal of Public Health*, *33*(Supplement 2), pp. ckad160–479.

Frenk, J., Chen, L. C., Chandran, L., Groff, E. O., King, R., Meleis, A. and Fineberg, H. V. (2022). Challenges and opportunities for educating health professionals after the COVID-19 pandemic. *The Lancet*, *400*(10362), pp. 1539–1556.

Han, Y., He, Y., Lyu, J., Yu, C., Bian, M. and Lee, L. (2020). Aging in China: Perspectives on public health. *Global Health Journal*, *4*(1), pp. 11–17.

Hardin, R. M. (2020). *Generation Z: Motivational needs of the newest workforce* (Doctoral dissertation, Northcentral University).

Hickson, S. V. (2024). Healthcare disparities. *Clinics in Integrated Care*, *22*, p. 100181.

Holland, J., Kingston, L., McCarthy, C., Armstrong, E., O'Dwyer, P., Merz, F. and McConnell, M. (2021). Service robots in the healthcare sector. *Robotics*, *10*(1), p. 47.

Hughes, G., Shaw, S. E. and Greenhalgh, T. (2020). Rethinking integrated care: A systematic hermeneutic review of the literature on integrated care strategies and concepts. *The Milbank Quarterly*, *98*(2), pp. 446–492.

International Labour Organization. (2022). *Getting Skills Right Equipping Health Workers with the Right Skills Skills Anticipation in the Health Workforce: Skills Anticipation in the Health Workforce.* OECD Publishing.

Karan, A., Negandhi, H., Hussain, S., Zapata, T., Mairembam, D., De Graeve, H., Buchan, J. and Zodpey, S. (2021). Size, composition, and distribution of health workforce in India: Why, and where to invest? *Human Resources for Health, 19,* pp. 1–14.

Khan, Z. F. and Alotaibi, S. R. (2020). Applications of artificial intelligence and big data analytics in m-health: A healthcare system perspective. *Journal of Healthcare Engineering,* pp. 1–15.

Kumar, P., Dwivedi, Y. K. and Anand, A. (2023). Responsible artificial intelligence (AI) for value formation and market performance in healthcare: The mediating role of patient's cognitive engagement. *Information Systems Frontiers, 25*(6), pp. 2197–2220.

Leerapan, B., Teekasap, P., Urwannachotima, N., et al. (2021). System dynamics modelling of health workforce planning to address future challenges of Thailand's Universal Health Coverage. *Human Resources of Health, 19*(31). https://doi.org/10.1186/s12960-021-00572-5

Leo, C. G., Sabina, S., Tumolo, M. R., Bodini, A., Ponzini, G., Sabato, E. and Mincarone, P. (2021). Burnout among healthcare workers in the COVID 19 era: A review of the existing literature. *Frontiers in Public Health, 9,* p. 750529.

Locke, R., Gambatese, M., Sellers, K., Corcoran, E. and Castrucci, B. C. (2022). Building a sustainable governmental public health workforce: A look at the millennial generation. *Journal of Public Health Management and Practice, 28*(1), pp. E198–E210.

Maeda, A. and Socha-Dietrich, K. (2021). *Skills for the Future Health Workforce: Preparing Health Professionals for People-centred Care.* OECD Health Working Papers, No. 124. Paris: OECD Publishing. https://dx.doi.org/10.1787/68fb5f08-en.

Myers, V. L. and Dreachslin, J. L. (2007). Recruitment and retention of a diverse workforce: Challenges and opportunities. *Journal of Healthcare Management, 52*(5), pp. 290–298.

Nazeha, N., Pavagadhi, D., Kyaw, B. M., Car, J., Jimenez, G. and Tudor Car, L. (2020). A digitally competent health workforce: Scoping review of educational frameworks. *Journal of Medical Internet Research, 22*(11), p. e22706.

Okoroafor, S. C., Asamani, J. A., Kabego, L., Ahmat, A., Nyoni, J., Millogo, J. J. S., Illou, M. M. A. and Mwinga, K. (2022). Preparing the health workforce for future public health emergencies in Africa. *BMJ Global Health, 7*(Supplement 1), p. e008327.

Pittman, P., Chen, C., Erikson, C., Salsberg, E., Luo, Q., Vichare, A., Batra, S. and Burke, G. (2021). Health workforce for health equity. *Medical Care, 59,* pp. S405–S408.

Ross, C. (2024). Building an interprofessional practice approach in a polytechnic institution beginning with health-care education and embracing the concept as an operational leadership imperative. *Journal of Innovation in Polytechnic Education, 6.*

Sarker, M. (2024). Revolutionizing healthcare: The role of machine learning in the health sector. *Journal of Artificial Intelligence General Science (JAIGS), 2*(1), pp. 35–48. ISSN: 3006-4023.

Sarker, S., Jamal, L., Ahmed, S. F. and Irtisam, N. (2021). Robotics and artificial intelligence in healthcare during COVID-19 pandemic: A systematic review. *Robotics and Autonomous Systems, 146,* p. 103902.

Stanford, F. C. (2020). The importance of diversity and inclusion in the healthcare workforce. *Journal of the National Medical Association, 112*(3), pp. 247–249.

Tariq, M. U. (2024). Advanced wearable medical devices and their role in transformative remote health monitoring. In *Transformative Approaches to Patient Literacy and Healthcare Innovation* (pp. 308–326). IGI Global.

Vesty, G., Jansson, M., Rana, T., Butler-Henderson, K. and Arabi, S. (2024). Workforce upskilling for value-based healthcare. In *Accounting for Healthcare* (pp. 91–102). Routledge.

Chapter 3

Equity, diversity and belonging in practice-based learning

Eric Nkansah Opoku and Jou Yin Teoh

CHAPTER OVERVIEW

Practice placement must consider how the diverse needs of students can be met to provide an environment that ensures equity, diversity and belonging. Diversity in characteristics of students can significantly affect their practice placement learning experiences. Diversity is multi-dimensional and includes race, disability, sexuality, gender, faith and belief, age, class, economic status and the intersections of these and other characteristics. Due to difference or perception of difference, students with diverse characteristics may experience oppression, marginalisation, alienation, discrimination, victimisation and/or harassment. This chapter aims to discuss issues of equity, diversity and belonging in practice-based learning and suggest practical ways to provide high-quality practice education that meets the needs of students from diverse backgrounds and/or those with diverse characteristics.

CHAPTER OBJECTIVES

The objectives of this chapter are the following.

- To examine how various aspects of diversity (such as race, disability, sexuality, gender, faith, age, class and economic status) influence the learning experiences of students during practice placements.
- To explore issues like oppression, marginalisation, alienation, discrimination, victimisation and harassment that students with diverse characteristics may face in practice placement settings.
- Discuss how the intersections of different characteristics (like race, disability, gender, etc.) create unique challenges and experiences for

---

DOI: 10.4324/9781003411765-3

students in practice placements, and how these intersections can be better understood and accommodated in practice education settings.

- Discuss strategies and approaches to foster an environment in practice placements that values and supports equity, diversity, inclusion and a sense of belonging among students.
- Offer practical recommendations and methods to enhance the quality of practice education so that it effectively meets the needs of students from diverse backgrounds and with diverse characteristics.

INTRODUCTION

In order to fulfil specified educational and regulatory requirements, allied health students are often required to complete a minimum number of hours of practice placement education in a variety of settings, including a range of age groups and conditions. For instance, in accordance with guidelines established by professional organisations like the World Federation of Occupational Therapists (WFOT) and the Royal College of Occupational Therapists (RCOT), occupational therapy students in the UK must complete a minimum of 1,000 hours of placement education across a variety of physical and mental health settings, serving a range of age groups and conditions (WFOT, 2016; RCOT, 2019). The extensive exposure that allied health professional students must receive provides them with a variety of skills, encourages interdisciplinary collaboration, improves cultural competency and trains well-rounded healthcare professionals, all of which contribute to safe and efficient practice in the allied health professions. These requirements ensure safe and successful practice in the allied health professions (Penman et al., 2023).

However, despite the diversity of practice settings and the variety of interactions, not all students may always encounter a conducive learning environment that actively promotes equity, diversity and belonging (EDB). There are still difficulties in enforcing these values through educational norms and accrediting standards. There are still obstacles that many students with varied backgrounds face that can obstruct their ability to be successful while on placement and to advance professionally. These obstacles, which can have a significant impact on their school experience and future job trajectories, range from covert biases to more overt forms of discrimination, victimisation and harassment.

In this chapter, we explore the essential components of EDB in practice-based learning settings. We will examine how universities and placement locations can foster a culture that actively embraces EDB to improve student learning and wellbeing. Regardless of a student's background or personal traits, the goal is to provide a practice education that is equitable and supportive for all. To that end, this chapter will also examine best practices and strategies to provide high-quality practice education that meets the needs of students from diverse backgrounds and/or with diverse characteristics.

USEFUL FRAMEWORKS FOR UNDERSTANDING EDB IN THE CONTEXT OF ALLIED HEALTH PROFESSION PRACTICE PLACEMENTS

Intersectionality

The concept of 'intersectionality' provides a critical lens for examining interpersonal interactions within practice learning contexts. These can include interactions between the student and service users, between practice educators or between other staff members on the placement site, as well as interactions between the various parties on site with the student as an observer. Originating from Kimberle Crenshaw, a Black feminist lawyer in the United States in 1989, intersectionality encapsulates the complex experiences of discrimination and workplace harassment faced by Black women that results from intersections between their racial and gender identities that defy neat compartmentalisation (Esposito and Evans-Winters, 2021).

An intersectional lens necessitates scrutinising the power relations between multiple structural dimensions such as national and racial or ethnic background, gender, age, language, socioeconomic status, legal status, and migration experience; considering how they influence one another in a variety of contexts; and deconstructing these dynamics in the process of addressing structural injustices and inequalities (Edwards and Esposito, 2020).

Although the term 'intersectionality' is modern, awareness of the concept pre-dates the term, as similar ideas have been articulated and developed by several scholars and activists identifying as women of colour from a variety of racial backgrounds. One key example is the concept of Triple Oppression advanced by Black feminist activists such as the Combahee River Collective (Jones, 1949; Davis, 1982). Over time, the concept has expanded to include other axes of power, and its use has been expanded into a range of political and academic fields including practice-based learning in the allied health professions (Cho et al., 2013; Edwards and Esposito, 2020; Teoh et al., 2024).

Curricular (in)congruence

In recent years, professional, statutory, and regulatory bodies (PSRBs) in the health and care professions have become more deliberate in attempts to EDB into academic curricula. Nonetheless, researchers have noted that it is common for knowledge gained by learners to be incongruent from intended curricula as far as such topics are concerned (Keyes et al., 2023). This disparity between learnt and intended curricula can be attributed to the influence of various factors sometimes collectively referred to as 'implicit curricula' which are not apparently explicit in academic curricula, and can include interpersonal interactions, institutional policies, organisational culture and/or wider contextual norms that shape learning environments (Hafferty, 1998; Council on Social Work Education, 2022)

Recognising that implicit curricula can both reinforce and undermine the explicit aspect of academic curricular goals (Bowl, 2005; Razack et al., 2014; Cheng and Yang, 2015; Murphy, 2019; Stergiopoulos et al., 2018; Council on Social Work Education, 2022; Webb et al., 2022), medical sociologist Frederic Hafferty (1998, p. 403) emphasised the need for attempts at curricular reform to be "undertaken with an eye on what students learn instead of what they are taught".

Even with the best of intentions, the implicit curriculum differs greatly between various learning environments and student demographics, complicating efforts to maintain curricular congruence (Cheng and Yang, 2015; Stergiopoulos et al., 2018; Webb et al., 2022; Fins and Del Pozo, 2011).

Consequently, curricular congruence can be difficult to maintain consistently across practice learning environments due to their highly variable and largely unstructured nature. Hence, we suggest that curricular incongruence should be acknowledged as an inevitable part of practice education in the health and care professions, and we suggest that this phenomenon has potential to be embraced as a valuable driver for change (Martimianakis et al., 2015; Abbaspour et al., 2022; Teoh et al., forthcoming).

PLANNING AND PREPARATION FOR PLACEMENT

University-based learning in the health and care professions serves as a foundation and gateway to prepare pre-qualification learners for practice education. Effective preparation before students go out on placement is essential to ensuring that principles of EDB are embedded from the outset.

What should the university do?

- **Preparing for informal and implicit learning**: Given that practice environments often rely on informal, self-directed learning, universities must equip students with strategies for navigating this implicit curriculum (Hafferty, 1998).
- **Feedback literacy**: This is crucial here. For feedback processes to be enhanced, students need both appreciation of how feedback can operate effectively and opportunities to use feedback within the placement setting (Nieminen and Carless, 2023). Students should be taught to actively seek, interpret and apply feedback to facilitate learning.
- **Peer-assisted learning**: Encouraging peer-assisted learning models within the classroom facilitates a culture of collaboration, mutual support and inclusion, helping students from diverse backgrounds feel less isolated.
- **Pre-placement preparation**: Students should be prepared for pre-placement visits or calls with practice educators to ease transition and clarify expectations.
- **Inclusive curriculum design**: Ensuring the curriculum includes modules that focus on health disparities, social determinants of health and the importance of culturally competent care. This ensures students are theoretically prepared to address and respect diversity in their practice placements. This approach will also help students understand a wide range of cultural competencies required in practice and promote an inclusive view of healthcare.
- **Disability services**: Disability services in universities play a key role in promoting EDB by identifying and addressing the needs of students with disabilities. These services proactively assess students' requirements and facilitate reasonable adjustments in academic and placement settings. The university placement coordinators need to collaborate with practice educators to discuss and implement necessary accommodations before student placements begin. This ensures that students with disabilities have equitable opportunities to succeed alongside their peers, helping to create an inclusive environment where all students feel valued, supported and empowered to thrive.
- **Comprehensive support profiles**: Beyond disability, university placement coordinators should discuss with placement educators support profiles including linguistic challenges and religious considerations – e.g., Ramadan, wearing of hijab and other unique requirements – to ensure equitable learning opportunities. These unique requirements should be discussed with placement educators before students start placement.
- **Placement allocation considerations**: When allocating placements to students, universities need to make consideration for protected characteristics,

such as disability or religious commitments (e.g., Ramadan). This could help reduce barriers.

- **Simulation placements and university clinics**: These controlled settings allow students to build confidence, address specific learning needs and develop skills in a supportive environment. Feedback mechanisms are particularly effective in these environments.
- **Practice educator training**: If possible, universities should provide structured training to practice educators, emphasising EDB principles to help create welcoming and inclusive environments for all students.

What should the practice setting do?

Practice settings must also commit to planning and preparing for EDB to ensure students feel welcomed and supported during practice placement. Key strategies include the following.

- **Practice educator training**: Practice educators should receive formal, ongoing training that addresses EDB values. This training must include practical tools for creating an inclusive learning environment, identifying unconscious biases and understanding how diverse characteristics intersect in students' experiences. Training can include case studies, role-playing scenarios, and reflective exercises to ensure placement educators are prepared to support a diverse student cohort effectively.
- **Onboarding programmes**: Placement settings should design comprehensive onboarding programmes that clearly communicate the setting's commitment to EDB. These programmes should include the following.

  - An introduction to the setting's policies on equity, diversity, anti-discrimination, and harassment.
  - Details on reporting mechanisms for concerns and incidents.
  - An overview of the organisational culture and EDB values.
  - Explicit instructions on how students can access support, including mentors, placement coordinator or external advocacy services.

  Onboarding sessions can also feature real-world examples of inclusive practices within the organisation to reinforce the importance of EDB principles in daily practice.
- **Pre-placement contact**: Pre-placement contact is vital for ensuring that students feel confident and supported as they begin their placements. Placement educators should engage in the following.

  - Schedule introductory calls or meetings to discuss expectations, learning goals and any specific accommodations or support needs.

- Provide a detailed overview of the placement setting, including cultural norms, dress codes, working hours and available resources.
- Encourage students to voice concerns or share personal considerations, such as religious practices, mental health needs or accessibility requirements.
- Use this opportunity to build rapport, foster trust and reassure students that their diversity will be respected and valued throughout the placement.

- **Policy transparency**: Placement settings must ensure students are aware of organisational policies that protect their rights and promote EDB. This can be achieved by the following.

  - Clearly communicating zero-tolerance policies for discrimination, harassment and victimisation.
  - Providing written guidelines that outline reporting procedures for grievances and detailing the support available to students who experience challenges.
  - Displaying EDB commitments visibly within the placement environment (e.g., posters, digital communications) to reinforce the organisation's culture of inclusion.
  - Sharing success stories and positive examples of inclusive practices to demonstrate real commitment to these policies.

BOX 3.1   PRACTICE EXAMPLES AND DESIGN FEATURES: PRE-PLACEMENT

Some placement designs require the following special pre-placement considerations to ensure EDB.

Long-arm supervision, role-emerging and technology-enabled placements: These placements often rely on virtual communication and technology, which can amplify issues such as communication breakdowns, feelings of isolation and digital inequities among students (Rafalow, 2020). Pre-placement preparation should include ensuring that all students have access to reliable technology, adequate training on digital tools and opportunities for regular virtual check-ins. Universities and placement providers must also recognise and address disparities in technological access, offering loan devices or additional support when necessary. Frequent virtual check-ins can also facilitate engagement and reduce feelings of disconnection during remote supervision.

Simulated placements and student-led clinics: In simulated environments or university-led clinics, universities have greater control over the structure and learning process (Bowman et al., 2019; Gunn et al., 2021). These placements provide an ideal opportunity to embed EDB principles through deliberate and structured approaches. Students can receive enhanced feedback and mentorship tailored to their unique needs, and simulation scenarios can be designed to reflect diverse patient demographics and culturally sensitive healthcare practices. This will prepare students for real-world diversity and also provides a safe, supportive space to address challenges they might encounter in other placements.

Interprofessional placements: Placements involving students from multiple professions can introduce challenges related to professional hierarchies and role clarity (Martin et al., 2022). Without preparation, students may experience exclusion or unequal opportunities based on perceived status of their professional group. Pre-placement strategies should include fostering a shared understanding of goals, responsibilities and mutual respect among all professions. Training sessions for educators and students can emphasise the value of interprofessional collaboration and reinforce EDB principles to prevent professional turf issues.

Public health and community-based placements: Placements in public health or community rehabilitation settings often involve engaging with underserved populations and addressing systemic health inequities (O'Mara-Eves et al., 2013). Students require pre-placement preparation that focuses on cultural competency, health disparities and the social determinants of health. Universities should equip students with the knowledge and skills to provide respectful, inclusive care, and encourage self-reflection to recognise and challenge personal biases. Placement providers should also offer culturally sensitive guidance to support students in navigating diverse and complex community contexts.

DURING PLACEMENT

The implementation phase is critical for ensuring that EDB principles translate into action during practice-based learning. Both universities and placement settings play important roles in facilitating a positive and inclusive experience for students.

What should the university do?

- **University representative contact personnel**: Assigning a dedicated university representative ensures students have access to direct support during placements. This representative serves as an advocate, mediator and liaison between students and practice settings to address challenges promptly.
- **Structured halfway calls or visits**: Incorporating midway check-ins between students, placement educators and university representatives ensures that issues are identified and addressed early. These calls facilitate feedback, provide reassurance and enhance student confidence.
- **Clear and accessible reporting processes**: Universities must establish transparent systems for reporting and addressing discrimination, harassment or other concerns. Confidential processes should be in place, ensuring that students feel safe and supported. Concerns reported should be subjected to timely investigations and appropriate actions taken. This will demonstrate the university's commitment to EDB principles and reassures students of support.
- **Peer and community support groups**: Universities can encourage students to form peer networks or community-based support groups during placements. These platforms provide safe spaces for sharing experiences, problem solving and building solidarity.
- **Check-ins with vulnerable groups**: Proactive contact with students who may experience additional challenges – such as students with disabilities, international students or those from marginalised backgrounds – will ensure their needs are continuously met.

What should the practice setting do?

- **Debriefing sessions**: Placement providers should offer regular debriefing sessions to provide students with safe spaces to reflect on their experiences, voice concerns and receive support. These sessions also allow practice educators to assess whether students feel included and supported.
- **Assessing belonging**: Educators should actively check in with students to gauge their sense of inclusion and belonging. This can include informal conversations or anonymous surveys. If any students express feeling isolated or excluded, immediate steps should be taken to address the issue, such as adjusting mentorship structures or reviewing team dynamics.
- **Mentorship and role modelling**: Providing mentors or role models who reflect diverse identities and experiences can significantly enhance students' sense of inclusion. Diverse mentors not only offer guidance and representation but also validate students' lived experiences. This is particularly beneficial

for students from marginalised or underrepresented backgrounds who may otherwise struggle to see themselves in leadership or professional roles.

- **Adapting workload and expectations**: Placement providers must demonstrate flexibility in accommodating students' specific needs. For instance, students observing religious practices, such as fasting during Ramadan, may benefit from adjusted schedules or lighter workloads at certain times. Similarly, students requiring reasonable adjustments due to disabilities or mental health needs should have tailored accommodations, such as assistive technology, regular breaks or workload adjustments.

BOX 3.2   PRACTICE EXAMPLES AND DESIGN FEATURES: DURING PLACEMENT

Some placement designs require special considerations during placement to ensure EDB:

Long-arm supervision, role-emerging and technology-enabled placements: Communication challenges must be addressed proactively. Providing structured, clear expectations and regular virtual meetings ensures students remain engaged. Digital tools, such as collaborative platforms and virtual mentorship, can facilitate interaction and minimise isolation.

Interprofessional placements: Educators must closely observe interprofessional dynamics to ensure collaboration remains equitable. Regular check-ins and facilitated discussions can address issues of professional hierarchy and encourage mutual respect among disciplines.

Public health and community-based placements: In underserved communities, placement educators must model culturally competent care and offer ongoing guidance to students, particularly around navigating challenges such as language barriers, socioeconomic disparities or stigma in healthcare access.

POST-PLACEMENT

Reflection and feedback are critical in the post-placement phase to drive continuous improvement and ensure EDB principles are upheld.

What should the university do?

- **Feedback mechanisms for continuous improvement**: Universities must gather feedback from students to assess their placement experiences, specifically relating to diversity, equity, inclusion, justice, accessibility and belonging (DEIJAB) challenges and successes. Feedback should be anonymous and inclusive, enabling students to share concerns safely. Diverse methods – such as anonymous surveys, reflective journals and facilitated focus groups – could be used to ensure that all voices are heard.

- **Using feedback for change**: Universities should analyse feedback to refine pre-placement preparation, identify systemic issues and work collaboratively with placement providers to improve future experiences. This process could include developing actionable plans and sharing aggregated feedback with placement providers to ensure transparency and accountability.
- **Post-placement reflection workshops**: Universities can facilitate structured workshops or focus groups that provide students with opportunities to share reflections on their experiences. These sessions help identify common challenges and successes, offering insights into improving EDB practices. Workshops can also include facilitated discussions led by EDB specialists or mentors to help students process their experiences.
- **Support for next steps**: For students who faced challenges, universities should provide post-placement support, such as counselling services, career advice or additional mentorship. This ensures students feel supported as they transition to the next stage of their education or career.

What should the practice setting do?

- **Evaluation and quality improvement**: Placement providers must establish formal processes to evaluate placements through student feedback. This could include both qualitative and quantitative methods – such as surveys, exit interviews and focus groups – to assess how effectively EDB principles were implemented and identify areas for improvement.
- **Encouraging honest feedback**: Creating a psychologically safe environment for students to share honest feedback, without fear of reprisal, is essential. Placement providers can use anonymous surveys or exit interviews to gather candid insights. Placement providers can use anonymous tools, such as secure online forms or written reflections, to mitigate fears of reprisal. Educators should explicitly emphasise to students that constructive feedback is valued and will lead to improvements.
- **Follow-up with students**: Placement providers should conduct follow-up conversations, either individually or as a group, to validate students' experiences and ensure that any unresolved challenges are addressed. These follow-ups demonstrate a genuine commitment to continuous improvement and allow educators to gauge the long-term impact of placements on students' professional growth.

- **Inclusive staff reflection**: Placement staff should engage in reflective practice to assess how effectively they upheld EDB principles during placements. Facilitated debriefing sessions for staff can help identify biases, gaps in knowledge or opportunities for improvement. This process promotes accountability and enhances educators' capacity to create inclusive learning environments.

BOX 3.3 PRACTICE EXAMPLES AND DESIGN FEATURES: POST-PLACEMENT

Some placement designs require the following special considerations post-placement to ensure EDB.

Long-arm supervision, role-emerging and technology-enabled placements: After remote placements, follow-up feedback should explore challenges such as digital access issues, feelings of isolation or communication barriers. This allows educators to implement improvements for future placements.

Simulated placements and student-led clinics: Structured debrief sessions encourage students to reflect on their learning outcomes and identify areas where further support or feedback may be needed. Educators can use this feedback to refine simulation activities for inclusivity.

Interprofessional placements: Post-placement debriefs involving all professions can address hierarchical challenges and promote collaboration. Joint reflections allow educators and students to explore shared goals, resolve conflicts and celebrate teamwork achievements.

Public health and community-based placements: Feedback mechanisms in these settings must assess whether students felt adequately prepared to work with underserved or diverse populations. Post-placement evaluations can highlight successes and inform ongoing strategies to improve culturally competent care delivery.

SUMMING UP WITH KEY PRINCIPLES

In practice-based learning, fostering EDB requires a coordinated effort between universities and practice settings. integrating EDB requires deliberate action at every stage of the placement, from preparation to post-placement reflection. This should be guided by a shared commitment to creating inclusive and supportive learning environments.

Preparation is a fundamental pillar in this process. Universities have the responsibility to equip students with the necessary skills, confidence and knowledge to navigate diverse and often informal learning environments. This preparation must include awareness of EDB principles, practical tools to manage challenges and opportunities to engage with diverse perspectives in a safe and constructive manner. Students who feel confident and equipped are more likely to engage actively and meaningfully in their practice placements.

Active partnerships between universities and practice settings are essential to embed EDB values throughout placement planning, implementation and evaluation. Collaborative relationships ensure that both institutions and placement settings are aligned in their commitment to fostering EDB. This partnership also enables the sharing of resources, training opportunities and best practices to enhance the overall placement experience.

Adopting student-centred approaches is another critical principle. Personalised support mechanisms are vital in addressing the unique needs of students from diverse backgrounds. When universities and placement setting acknowledge and accommodate individual differences, they can ensure that all students feel respected, included and empowered to succeed. Personalised support may include tailored adjustments for students with disabilities and/or religious commitments, linguistic support for non-native speakers or mentorship for underrepresented groups.

Feedback and continuous improvement form the backbone of sustainable EDB practices. Universities and placement settings must establish robust systems for gathering feedback from students and stakeholders to assess the success of EDB initiatives. This feedback should inform ongoing refinements to policies, training and placement structures, ensuring that EDB practices remain responsive to evolving student needs and societal changes.

Cultural competence is integral to preparing students to deliver inclusive and respectful care. Embedding cultural competency within academic curricula and practice education enables students to engage thoughtfully with diverse patient populations, address health disparities and contribute to equitable healthcare delivery. Students who develop cultural competence are better positioned to foster trust, respect and understanding in their professional interactions.

Integrating these principles (preparation, active partnership, student-centred approaches, feedback and continuous improvement, and cultural competence) into every stage of the placement process will enable universities and practice settings to create environments where all students – regardless of their background or personal characteristics – feel valued, supported and empowered to thrive. This commitment will enrich the educational journey of students and strengthens the capacity of the health and care professions to deliver equitable and inclusive services to diverse communities.

REFERENCES

Abbaspour, H., Moonaghi, H. K., Kareshki, H. and Esmaeili, H. (2022). Positive consequences of the hidden curriculum in undergraduate nursing education: An integrative review. *Iranian Journal of Nursing and Midwifery Research*, *27*(3), pp. 169–180.

Bowl, M. (2005). Valuing diversity in the social science curriculum. *LATISS: Learning and Teaching in the Social Sciences*, *2*(2), pp. 121–136. https://doi.org/10.1386/ltss.2.2.121/1

Bowman, A., Harreveld, R. B. and Lawson, C. (2019). A discussion paper on key issues impacting the sonographer workforce in Australia. *Sonography*, *6*(3), pp. 110–118. https://doi.org/10.1002/sono.12198

Cheng, L. F. and Yang, H. C. (2015). Learning about gender on campus: An analysis of the hidden curriculum for medical students. *Medical Education*, *49*(3), pp. 321–331.

Cho, S., Crenshaw, K. W. and McCall, L. (2013). Toward a field of intersectionality studies: Theory, applications, and praxis. *Signs: Journal of Women in Culture and Society*, *38*(4), pp. 785–810.

Council on Social Work Education. (2022). *Educational policy and accreditation standards for baccalaureate and master's social work programs*. Available at: https://www.cswe.org/getmedia/bb5d8afe7680-42dc-a332-a6e6103f4998/2022-EPAS.pdf

Davis, A. (1982). *Women, Race, and Class*. London: The Women's Press.

Edwards, E. B. and Esposito, J. (2020). *Intersectional Analysis as a Method to Analyze Popular Culture Clarity in the Matrix*. Routledge.

Esposito, J. and Evans-Winters, V. (2021). *Introduction to Intersectional Qualitative Research*. SAGE Publications, Incorporated.

Fins, J. J. and Del Pozo, P. R. (2011). The hidden and implicit curricula in cultural context: New insights from Doha and New York. *Academic Medicine*, *86*(3), pp. 321–325.

Gunn, T., Rowntree, P., Starkey, D. and Nissen, L. (2021). The use of virtual reality computed tomography simulation within a medical imaging and a radiation therapy undergraduate programme. *Journal of Medical Radiation Sciences*, *68*(1), pp. 28–36. https://doi.org/10.1002/jmrs.436

Hafferty, F. W. (1998). Beyond curriculum reform. *Academic Medicine*, *73*(4), pp. 403–407. https://doi.org/10.1097/00001888-199804000-00013

Jones, C. (1949). We seek full equality for women. *Reprinted in Viewpoint Magazine* [online]. (Accessed April 14 2025).

Keyes, T. S., Hendrix, E., Tecle, A., Andino, C., Bitters, B., Carter, R., Koelling, E., Ortiz, E., Sanchez, M., Ota, I. and Gringeri, C. (2023). "We wonder if white peers even want to understand": Social work students' experiences of the culture of human interchange. *Journal of Social Work Education*, *59*(1), pp. 229–242.

Martimianakis, M. A. T., Michalec, B., Lam, J., Cartmill, C., Taylor, J. S. and Hafferty, F. W. (2015). Humanism, the hidden curriculum, and educational reform: A scoping review and thematic analysis. *Academic Medicine*, *90*(11), pp. S5–S13.

Martin, P., Hill, A., Ford, M., Barnett, T., Graham, N. and Argus, G. (2022). A novel interprofessional education and supervision student placement model: Student and clinical educator perspectives and experiences. *International Journal of Environmental Research and Public Health*, *19*(17), pp. 107–134.

Murphy, M. (2019). Teaching and learning about sexual diversity within medical education: The promises and pitfalls of the informal curriculum. *Sexuality Research and Social Policy*, *16*(1), pp. 84–99.

Nieminen, J. H. and Carless, D. (2023). Feedback literacy: A critical review of an emerging concept. *Higher Education*, *85*(6), pp. 1381–1400.

O'Mara-Eves, A., Brunton, G., McDaid, D., Oliver, S., Kavanagh, J., Jamal, F., Matosevic, T., Harden, A. and Thomas, J. (2013). Community engagement to reduce inequalities in health: A systematic review, meta-analysis, and economic analysis. *Public Health Research*, *1*(4), pp. 1–526.

Penman, M., Raymond, J., Kumar, A., Liang, R. Y., Sundar, K. and Thomas, Y. (2023). Allied health professions accreditation standards for work integrated learning: A document analysis. *International Journal of Environmental Research and Public Health*, *20*(15), p. 6478.

Rafalow, M. H. (2020). *Digital Divisions: How Schools Create Inequality in the Tech Era*. University of Chicago Press.

Razack, S., Lessard, D., Hodges, B. D., Maguire, M. H. and Steinert, Y. (2014). The more it changes; the more it remains the same: A foucauldian analysis of Canadian policy documents relevant to student selection for medical school. *Advances in Health Sciences Education*, *19*, pp. 161–181.

Royal College of Occupational Therapists. (2019). *Learning and Development Standards for Pre-Registration Education* (Revised ed. 2019). London: Royal College of Occupational Therapists.

Stergiopoulos, E., Fernando, O. and Martimimianakis, M. A. (2018). "Being on both sides": Canadian medical students' experiences with disability, the hidden curriculum, and professional identity construction. *Academic Medicine*, *93*(10), pp. 1550–1559.

Teoh, J. Y., Lai, S. M., Sudhir, G., Fatimehin, M., Otermans, P., Horton, A., Saunders, E., Ludhra, G. and Barbosa Bouças, S. (forthcoming). Colour-evasive racial ideologies underpinning the hidden curriculum of a majority-minority occupational therapy school in London, England: An analysis of minoritised undergraduate students' experiences. *Oxford Review of Education*, pp. 1–19.

Webb, J., Arthur, R., McFarlane-Edmond, P., Burns, T. and Warren, D. (2022). An evaluation of the experiences of the hidden curriculum of Black and minority ethnic undergraduate health and social care students at a London university. *Journal of Further and Higher Education*, *46*(3), pp. 312–326.

World Federation of Occupational Therapists. (2016). *Minimum Standards for the Education of Occupational Therapists* (Revised ed. 2016. [s.l.]). World Federation of Occupational Therapists.

Chapter 4

Peer-assisted learning
Same-level and near-peer approaches within placements

Emma Green, Merrolee Penman and Jennie Brentnall

CHAPTER OVERVIEW

This chapter introduces peer-assisted learning (PAL) as an effective educational approach to enhance practice-based learning, incorporating both same-level peer learning and near-peer mentoring (NPM). PAL is a widely recognised and valued evidence-based approach in allied health education that can support learning in varied placement models. As a contemporary method to optimise learning opportunities and support learner success, it can function as a core component of practice-based learning that complements placement models discussed in this book. This chapter outlines the essential elements of PAL, and how same-level and near-peer approaches facilitate learning. It also summarises and evaluates the evidence base for PAL, with a focus on allied health placements. Evidence-based, real-world practice examples and expertise are distilled into practical principles for designing, planning, implementing and evaluating PAL. Practice examples are provided to illustrate applications of PAL, showcasing its use in routine placement offerings in a tertiary teaching hospital, rural peer-assisted learning clinic, and quality improvement of primary care services.

CHAPTER OBJECTIVES

The objectives of this chapter are the following.

- Provide an overview of PAL as an educational approach to practice-based learning.
- Summarise the evidence base related to PAL, with a focus on allied health.

DOI: 10.4324/9781003411765-4

- Outline practical principles for designing, planning, implementing and evaluating PAL in placements in allied health practice settings.
- Provide real-world examples to illustrate the design and implementation of PAL in placements in a range of settings.

INTRODUCTION

PAL is an educational approach rooted in contemporary adult learning theories. It serves as an umbrella term for various methods whereby peers learn with and from each other (Boud, 2001). Specifically, PAL has been defined as "a social practice of mutually beneficial personal and professional development among learners interacting as status equals, characterized by safety, comfort, motivation through relevance, and intellectual risk-taking" (Callese et al., 2019, p. 12). It encompasses both peer-to-peer learning among students at the same level and NPM between learners one or more academic years apart (Penman et al., 2024, p. 2). In practice-based learning, PAL typically involves pairs or small groups of 4–6 learners, though larger groups are possible. Regardless of whether learners are at the same level, in near-peer relationships or both, social practices of collaboration between learners sets PAL apart from traditional one-to-one apprenticeship models of practice-based learning.

PAL aligns with educational theories in higher education that emphasise collaborative, inquiry-based, group and student-facilitated approaches to learning (Tai et al., 2021). To facilitate PAL in the context of practice-based learning, a practice educator intentionally supports learners to engage in a structured and deliberate collaboration that is aligned with learning outcomes to enhance the learning experience (Beveridge and Pentland, 2020; Pope et al., 2023; Penman et al., 2024). The practice educator is instrumental in designing the placement model, guiding the collaborative learning process that supports students' development of confidence in their growing knowledge and skills (Markowski et al., 2021). This marks a shift from traditional, instructor-led placement models to a more facilitative, student-centred approach to learning.

PAL has evolved into a recognised approach in pre-registration practice-based learning across health and social care professions (Brierley et al., 2022). It is applied successfully across a variety of settings, including both public and private healthcare; role-emerging settings including charities, non-government organisations or social enterprises; research; and leadership project placements.

Providing an effective, flexible and adaptable model, PAL has firmly established itself as a valuable and complementary approach across a diverse range of practice settings (Penman et al., 2024).

LEARNING THEORIES UNDERPINNING PEER-ASSISTED LEARNING

PAL is based on social learning theories. These posit that learning is inherently social, with knowledge acquisition shaped by the interactions we have with one another (Boud, 2001) and our social contexts and environments (Patton et al., 2018). Lave and Wenger's (1991, p. 45) concept of "communities of practice" emphasises that practice settings each possess their own unique understandings and traditions. In these practice settings, learners transition gradually from observing to actively engaging in tasks, demonstrating their competency through social engagement and collaborative work in authentic practice environments (Wenger, 1998). Of relevance to PAL, in these practice environments, learning occurs not only between educators and learners, but also among learners (Lave and Wenger, 1991; Boud and Middleton, 2003). Learners achieve this by assisting each other, solving problems, discussing situations and needs, exploring, bouncing ideas with and off each other, and providing peer feedback (Palsson et al., 2021). These peer interactions are central to a rich PAL practice-based learning experience.

A key enabler of PAL is that learners share social roles (social congruence) and comparable academic backgrounds (cognitive congruence) as compared with their educators (Loda et al., 2019). This common ground fosters supportive learning environments, as peers communicate in a shared language that aids in clarifying expectations and experiences, and provides informal support – often more effectively than that offered by a more experienced practice educator (Loda et al., 2019). Each learner has their own "zone of proximal development" representing the knowledge, and skills just beyond their capabilities (Vygotsky, 1978, p. 86). With the support of a peer or near peer with slightly greater capability in a specific area, a learner can be supported to achieve their learning objectives. The roles may then be reversed in another area of knowledge or skill. In a typical PAL placement – especially in near-peer mentoring where one student is more experienced and there is a "more capable other" – the zone of proximal development (ZPD) thereby becomes a powerful driver of collaborative learning. These dynamics of social learning, combined with a safe space for learners to ask questions and be curious, are vital to the success of a PAL placement.

EVIDENCE BASE FOR PEER-ASSISTED LEARNING ON PLACEMENT

The evidence base for PAL placements has developed greatly in the last 30 years. Compared with medicine (Brierley et al., 2022) and nursing (Carey et al., 2018), where PAL and NPM models have been widely utilised in both academic coursework and placement settings, there are fewer studies to inform the design of PAL and NPM in allied health–specific placements. There is also an ongoing allegiance to the one supervisor/one student model of placement in some areas of allied health (Pope et al., 2023). Nonetheless, there has been sufficient research to enable several allied health–focused systematic reviews. Same-level PAL systematic reviews include those by Briffa and Porter (2013) and Sevenhuysen et al. (2017) for allied health students, with Secomb (2008) and Markowski et al. (2021) including both allied health and nursing students, and both PAL and NPM placement types. A recent review by Pope et al. (2023) of allied health studies included PAL as one of the placement models but did not distinguish between same or different level peers, while only one systematic review focusing on NPM allied health placements (Penman et al., 2024) has been located.

The evidence base demonstrates that students generally value PAL placements as enabling their personal and professional growth, skill acquisition (Briffa and Porter, 2013; Penman et al., 2024; Pope et al., 2023; Secomb, 2008) and confidence (Secomb, 2008). Students and/or their educators identify enhanced opportunities to develop students' autonomy, along with their problem-solving and professional reasoning (Pope et al., 2023; Secomb, 2008). Other areas of student development include reflective practice (Briffa and Porter, 2013; Pope et al., 2023), along with developing skills such as time management, teamwork and effective communication (Markowski et al., 2021; Penman et al., 2024: Pope et al., 2023; Sevenhuysen, 2017). PAL placements also provide a level of emotional or peer support (Pope et al., 2023), with students using each other as learning resources (Briffa and Porter, 2013). PAL placements may also promote students' stress management and health (Jassim et al., 2022) and evaluative judgement (Tai et al., 2016), although these outcomes have not been investigated specifically with allied health students.

Interestingly, some studies have identified differences in how senior students engage in the learning of their junior peers. For example, the study by Hari et al. (2022) of radiological students, whereby near-peer mentors were observed to spend more time on exploring learning gaps and establishing a safe learning climate compared to their educators focus on skill acquisition; or Penman et al.

(2021), whereby senior peers provided more detailed feedback than the junior students' educators. Finally, NPM placements may also provide senior students with inspiration to become educators through the development of their educator skills (Markowski et al., 2021; Penman et al., 2024; Secomb, 2008).

While fewer studies have explored the value of PAL for educators, it is generally perceived positively (Briffa and Porter, 2013; Penman et al., 2024). Outcomes reported for educators have included clinical educator skill development and – for some – productivity benefits (Penman et al., 2024; Pope et al., 2023; Sevenhuysen et al., 2013), although others have reported increased time commitments (Markowski et al., 2021). Educators have also identified some concerns with PAL models, including managing challenges such as differing student personalities and capabilities (Markowski et al., 2021; Pope et al., 2023), and concerns about the quality of the learning experienced between the peers, although this is less of a concern in NPM PAL, and fewer opportunities to assess each student in their own right (Pope et al., 2023). In addition, challenges with sufficient caseload could impact on student learning (Pope et al., 2023).

Few studies have investigated the impact of PAL with service users, and to date those that have report from the supervisor or student perspective, identifying that PAL/NPM models have improved service users' care and progression through continuity of services (Penman et al., 2024). While some studies report service users' willingness to support student learning (Penman et al., 2024; Pope et al., 2023; Secomb, 2008), others interestingly did not recognise the primary role students had had in their service provision (Penman et al., 2024).

The evidence base also speaks to the enablers and barriers to the successful adoption of PAL. It is essential that educators are introduced to strategies that will support PAL (Sevenhuysen, 2017). Similarly, students also need to be oriented to their roles in supporting each other's learning (Sevenhuysen, 2017), especially given that most students' experiences are still likely to have been in one-supervisor/one-student placement models (Pope et al., 2023). Consideration also needs to be given to space requirements (Briffa and Porter, 2013) and the educator's perceived increase in administration, as well as scheduling group and/ or individual supervision, and the assessment of student performance (Markowski et al., 2021; Pope et al., 2023). Other disadvantages may include managing student relationships and differing competence levels (Briffa and Porter, 2013; Markowski et al., 2021; Secomb, 2008), as well as ensuring that there is sufficient caseload for all students (Briffa and Porter, 2013; Secomb, 2008; Pope et al., 2023).

The benefits of PAL and NPM are noted in Box 4.1.

```
┌──────────────────────────────────────────────────────────────┐
│           BOX 4.1   BENEFITS OF PAL AND NPM                    │
│                                                                │
│                         LEARNERS                               │
│                                                                │
│  • Enables personal and professional growth, skill acquisition │
│    and confidence.                                             │
│  • Supports students' development of professional reasoning    │
│    and reflective practice.                                    │
│  • Develops skills such as communication, teamwork and         │
│    leadership.                                                 │
│  • Develops students' knowledge and skills for a future        │
│    educator role.                                              │
│  • Provides opportunities for support (emotional/learning)     │
│    from peers.                                                 │
│                                                                │
│                    PRACTICE EDUCATORS                          │
│                                                                │
│  • Further develop educators' skills in the facilitation of    │
│    learning.                                                   │
│  • Opportunities for professional development.                 │
│  • Can enhance productivity of the educator and/or service,    │
│    allowing for some relieve time.                             │
│                                                                │
│                      SERVICE USERS                             │
│                                                                │
│  • Perceived improvement in continuity of care.                │
│  • Care received may be more comprehensive.                    │
│                                                                │
│                        UNIVERSITY                              │
│                                                                │
│  • PAL and NPM may facilitate an increase in placement         │
│    capacity.                                                   │
│  • For those experiencing NPM placements, senior students      │
│    may be more inspired and feel more confident in adopting    │
│    the educator role.                                          │
└──────────────────────────────────────────────────────────────┘
```

DESIGN PRINCIPLES FOR PAL

PAL offers a flexible, student-centred approach to learning, distinct from traditional placement structures and supervision models (Pope et al., 2023). It provides a range of opportunities for enhancing placements without necessarily adding to workload, but maximising its benefits for learners, patients/service users, practice educators and services, and higher education institutes requires thoughtful design (Penman et al., 2024). This section outlines the essential design principles to help you create effective PAL placements, guiding you from pre-placement planning through to post-placement review and reflection. Key points are summarised in Table 4.1 and detailed in what follows.

Table 4.1 Design principles for peer-assisted learning

Rationale for choice of PAL	• Design to specifically facilitate collaborative learning that is targeted at achieving specific learning outcomes, e.g., developing, problem solving, clinical reasoning or evaluative judgement; developing teamwork, leadership skills or confidence in emerging competence; developing skills in the education of others.
Approach to supervision	• Practice educators need to develop a safe and supportive space for collaborative learning, and aspects of the role and structure of supervision need to be considered. • The relationship within and between peers needs to be explicitly considered to ensure alignment with learning outcomes and supported by supervision structure. • Planning to set ground rules and working arrangement within and between peers and supervisors is key.
Mode of delivery and learning	• Main considerations relate to whether the placement is set up as a fully integrated PAL placement or designated PAL activity for specific tasks throughout the week.
Planning and preparation	• Planning needs to consider the learning outcomes desired (rationale); the level of PAL, either full or designated activities (mode); and types of relationships between peers (supervision structures). • Practical planning relating to sufficient induction to model of placement and scheduling time initially and as placement progresses. • Practical planning required in relation to service user–related collaborative activities and considerations of space and technologies to support this.
Implementing placement	• Nurture collaborative learning from the very beginning. • Shift over time from directing learners to enabling their collaboration with appropriate review and feedback particularly with near peers whereby senior students take lead and guide junior students on identified areas. • Monitor and assist learners to manage relative and total workloads, navigate interpersonal relations, and solve problems collaboratively. • Adjust strategies to individual needs and differences in performance between learners.
Learner diversity, equity and inclusion	• Foster inclusion and belonging through effective collaboration and creating safe space with a clear approach to peer support and shared learning.

Table 4.1 Continued

	• Utilise the relative proximity of peers to each other and opportunities to access multiple perspectives to increase feelings of inclusion, developing cultural capabilities and increased understanding working with service users, colleagues and communities from diverse backgrounds. • Facilitating learning between peers with different learning needs and preferences (developing professional skills for all).
Considerations for learner feedback, assessment and evaluation	• Capitalise on opportunities for multi-directional (or multi-source feedback) to develop students' evaluative judgement and inform assessment for and of learning. • Ensure that students are supported to develop skills in feedback conversations, understanding that an honest and compassionate approach – supported by observations – is usually appreciated. • Practice educator feedback should be informal and formal, and focus on individual and collaborative aspects. • Practice educator has overall responsibility for summative assessment informed by feedback from all key individuals.
Post-placement	• Review against the placement aims. • Include the perspectives of all stakeholder groups. • Specifically consider the achievement of intended PAL outcomes and the knowledge, skills and attributes promoted or hindered by PAL.
Resources, funding, capacity, hidden costs	• Resource-efficient model that has the potential to increase capacity only if designed well to make use of collaborative learning rather than multiply the supervision of individuals. • Initial investment is needed to develop the model and resources to support peer collaborative learning.

Rationale for PAL

The key design decision for adopting PAL – for all or part of a placement – is determining how bringing peers together to learn with and from each other can help achieve the intended learning outcomes. PAL involves deliberately bringing learners together – either in person or online – in pairs or small groups, with a clear focus on collaborative learning (Sevenhuysen et al., 2017). This is different from simply co-locating students together without a structured shared learning goal (Penman et al., 2024). For example, PAL might have learning pairs working together throughout the whole placement on tasks like information gathering, assessment or designing and implementing interventions with service users, helping students develop both task-related and interpersonal skills. Alternatively, groups or pairs of students may collaborate on quality improvement projects, honing their problem-solving and teamwork abilities. For NPM, the deliberate design would include first ensuring the senior student was competent in some aspects of practice, then developing their skills in how to support or facilitate the learning of a junior peer – thus developing their educator skills in preparation for a future student supervisor role.

PAL offers flexibility and innovation, making it adaptable to a broad range of learning outcomes and placement needs. When designing PAL for a placement, the reason for choosing PAL should be led by the intended learning outcomes that are typically communicated by the university, but often individual students will have their own areas for development within the broader learning outcomes. University staff will usually provide practice educators support with this planning related to aligning learning outcomes and collaborative learning activities on request.

- **To develop autonomy and professional reasoning**: You might arrange for the PAL students to manage a small caseload including review of file, information gathering, assessment and/or intervention planning, with the students discussing their reasoning for their actions with supervisor and/or other students.
- **To develop communication and team working skills**: Tasks might involve working in pairs on a shared project to develop team working skills or peer observation of interpersonal skills with service users and then provide peer feedback.
- **To develop feedback and evaluative judgement skills**: Through practice or project tasks, learners may self-assess their skills or use peer assessment and feedback to help make judgements about their own abilities against given standards to support their development of evaluative judgement.
- **To develop supervisor/educator skills, leadership and delegation skills**: NPM could be used to guide the senior student to role model practice skills and then for them to support junior student to develop these skills in their own practice whilst being supported by a relatable peer. In turn, this develops many skills in the senior student, including those specific to the educator role.

In a PAL placement, you may focus on one or a combination of these areas as part of the intended learning from the placement. Having clarity regarding what you hope to achieve by designing collaborative learning experiences then helps direct how you plan, implement, assess and evaluate the placement as noted in subsequent sections.

Approach to supervision

Designing and delivering PAL requires the practice educator to thoughtfully plan, create and guide opportunities for peers to collaborate, enabling skill development and mutual learning. This approach affects both the supervisor's role and the supervision structure.

Considerations for the structure of supervision

Implementing PAL successfully starts with setting up clear expectations for roles and relationships, especially since students may be new to or even unsure about the benefits of this collaborative approach. An initial consideration is your aim for having the peers learn together, along with creating clear expectations for their working relationship between each other and with you as their practice educator. Following are some models of how to set up the working relationship within and between same or near-peer learners.

- **Equal collaborators**: For example, to meet the learning outcomes, it is best that the learners work as equal contributors to all collaborative learning activities sharing responsibility, balancing teamwork and mutual responsibility.
- **Parallel contributors**: This approach allows for addressing individual learning outcomes within collaborative tasks by facilitating learners to work in parallel and take responsibility for certain parts of an overall tasks. This may allow them to meet individual learning needs within a collaborative learning space.
- **Hierarchical relationship**: In a near-peer scenario, the peer relationship may be more hierarchical, where one or more senior students take the lead on discrete tasks to support one or more junior student(s) learning, e.g., undertaking initial information gathering/interviews, making phone calls to set up appointments or undertaking part of an intervention with guidance to ensure safety of service user and student.

As a supervisor, having clarity of these relationships aligned with intended learning outcomes for each student helps you set up appropriate role expectations of the learners and clarity on your role and structures to put in place as a supervisor.

In planning supervision for successful PAL placements, practice educators and learners should do the following.

- **Establish ground rules**: Agree on conduct and participation rules to foster collaboration and achieve learning outcomes.

- **Define roles and boundaries**: Clarify responsibilities, including addressing learning support, resolving issues and assessing capabilities.
- **Promote a supportive team environment**: Encourage feedback, recognise strengths and prioritise collaboration over competition.
- **Incorporate joint and individual supervision**: Use joint sessions for shared expectations and reflections, alongside individual guidance tailored to individual learning needs.
- **Develop evaluative judgement through supervision**: Support students in identifying strengths, setting goals and achieving shared objectives through self-assessment, peer learning, reflection and feedback.

Considerations for the supervisor role

The practice educator's role in PAL is to create structured opportunities whereby peers can learn collaboratively, with activities tailored to offer the right level of challenge. This involves monitoring and supporting both individual progress and group dynamics, and evaluating student knowledge and skills against learning outcomes (see the following section on feedback and assessment). It also requires the practice educator to create a safe space to nurture and facilitate learning within and between learners and be open to ongoing monitoring of the structure to ensure that the right level of challenge and arrangements are achieving the intended learning opportunities.

To facilitate this practice, educators need to consider the following.

- **Balance challenge and support**: Encourage idea-sharing and planning while guiding students on when to check reasoning for their actions with the supervisor. This can be supported by providing risk-assessed tasks matched to their level of skill to support growth and development and ensure the 'right level of challenge' in a safe space.
- **Foster independence**: Use intentional role modelling to build evaluative skills and reduce reliance on guidance, freeing educators' time for other tasks.
- **Prioritising collaboration and feedback**: Focus learning on teamwork, interpersonal skills and clinical reasoning suitable for the students' learning level and planned learning outcomes.

Mode of delivery

PAL – being defined by peer interactions, shared learning and collaboration – can be delivered in multiple modes: in person, online or and hybrid (see Chapter 6). PAL also lends itself to supporting and enhancing student experiences where there is not a practice educator on-site, including rural and remote locations where there may be additional isolation. Therefore, PAL can often be a key design feature of making long-arm supervision more effective (see Chapter 5).

Whether in person, online or hybrid, the main emphasis in PAL is on creating a shared safe space to learn together, share work and provide opportunities for feedback and discussion within and between peers, as well as with and from the practice educator. To this end, one of the main decisions for the mode of delivery is considering which of the following the placement will be.

- **Fully integrated PAL**: PAL could be woven throughout the experience, allowing students to collaborate on most tasks – manage relative and total workloads, navigate interpersonal relations and collaborate on project work. This model provides ongoing peer support and enables consistent opportunities for joint problem solving and feedback.
- **Designated PAL activities**: PAL could also be limited to specific components, such as leading a client group or working on a project one or two days per week. This allows students to concentrate on collaborative skills in structured settings and provides the opportunity to focus on independent work during other times.

This level of PAL will be directed by the learning you wish to achieve and will have a direct influence on how you plan and implement the placement.

Planning and preparation

In planning for successful PAL placements, practice educators need to have not just a commitment to facilitating learning within and between peers but also effective understanding of the design and implementation of PAL placements. Practice educators may need to invest time in their own learning and understanding of how to design and deliver a PAL placement.

Once the rationale for PAL aligned to learning outcomes is agreed, levels of PAL – either fully or designated activities – established and the relationship within and between learners and their supervisor developed, as outlined in the previous subsections, attention can turn to the placement and PAL structure to ensure sufficient planning for how the placement will be delivered. The following are some practical considerations to be considered in how to provide induction and manage learner's time.

- **Support placement setup**: Provide guidance and a clear induction to ease learner anxiety and clarify expectations for working and learning in a PAL placement.
- **Establish a clear schedule**: Initially, timetable collaborative learning, independent tasks and educator meetings to set clear expectations.
- **Practice educator initially lead planning**: The practice educator should initially lead scheduling based on learning goals and opportunities within the context, as they have knowledge of the intended learning outcomes and learning plan.
- **Plan to encourage learner autonomy**: For longer placements and appropriate to assessed level of skill, the practice educator should transition scheduling responsibilities to learners to promote independence.

Other practical consideration in planning relates to the learning activities themselves, particularly if these are related to service-user contact. The following practical aspects should be considered.

- **Provide sufficient space and technology**: Ensure physical or technological support for multiple learners without overcrowding or overwhelming situations.
- **Respect service-user preferences**: Ask service users their comfort level with (multiple) learner involvement, rather than making assumptions.
- **Optimise peer support to minimise practice educator presence**: Use risk-assessed learning activities with peers to minimise the need for practice educators' presence while keeping support accessible, e.g., available in the next room or next cubicle, or available by phone, text or pager as appropriate.
- **Optimise learning through planning and debriefing**: When learners cannot all be present with a service user, utilise planning, briefing before and debriefing after sessions to involve all learners in learning and reflection. This time for thinking and reflection can be as valuable as the direct contact time.

Implementing placement

A key to PAL success is fostering collaborative learning from the start by creating a culture of safety, support and clear expectations. Well-planned timetables provide reassurance, helping students feel secure in the new learning environment. Early on, ground rules should be negotiated and learners' knowledge and experiences should be acknowledged to ensure a sense of belonging and respect. Plan for the role to shift as the placement progresses primarily to one of facilitating the learning rather than being the provider of the learning. As the placement progresses, the practice educator's role shifts from directing learners to enabling collaboration, reviewing work, providing feedback and boosting learners' confidence in their individual and collective abilities. This will be supported by clear implementation of the supervision structures and approaches described previously.

The potential for interpersonal mismatches, conflict and negative competition between the students remains a concern to practice educators, although it is rare with active management strategies. Some strategies that can be considered are the following.

- **Reducing tension**: Time apart and a mix of individual and collaborative tasks can help manage relationships.
- **Developing workplace skills**: Encourage professional sharing and management of thoughts, feelings and knowledge. This helps develop team working skills, conflict management and work-readiness skills for future practice.

Another concern of educators is the management of the (relative) underperformance of a student and the impacts that has on PAL during placements. In practice, it is essential to monitor and adjust learning strategies throughout any placement to ensure ongoing effectiveness. The strategies to adjust learning to address underperformance are the same as in any placement, even in a situation when a senior near-peer learner is having difficulty, then the model can still be supportive. Some practical strategies to help an underperforming learner include the following.

- **Peer support for underperformance**: Peers can support learning through modelling, feedback and collaborative problem solving. Junior peers can help senior students by asking questions and exploring practice skills and concepts.
- **Clear practice educator roles**: Educators must maintain clear roles in providing additional support and assessing student competence. Ensure that learners understand the educator's role in guiding and evaluating their progress.
- **Adjust collaboration levels**: Adjust the extent of collaboration depending on differences in learners' capabilities. Ensure that all learners, regardless of their performance level, have opportunities suited to their current and emerging abilities.

Learner diversity, equity and inclusion

Well-planned and proficiently facilitated PAL can foster inclusion and belonging for all parties, increasing the equitable access to opportunities and outcomes for diverse learners. When peer relationships are set up well to enable safety and collaboration, the closer proximity of peers to each other than to educators can increase feelings of inclusion for marginalised learners. A well-designed PAL can achieve the following.

- **Address and accommodate for diverse learning needs**: Within PAL, you can have access to multiple perspectives, explanations and feedback that may help to meet varied learning needs. Practice educators can make accommodations – such as dedicated reflection time – which benefit all learners without disadvantaging others.
- **Promote and support greater understanding and inclusion**: PAL provides opportunity for peers to understand and apply accommodations, expanding their understanding of how accommodations can be effective to meet the needs of all. Through collaboration, diverse learners can share experiences, fostering respect and understanding of diversity, equity and inclusion.
- **Develop cultural capabilities**: Prolonged collaboration between learners from diverse backgrounds can lead to understandings of what informs different perspectives, thus enhancing the student's capabilities for their future practice with diverse service users, colleagues and communities.

Considerations for learner feedback, assessment and evaluation

As in all placement experiences, feedback is an integral tool to support learners' growth and development throughout PAL. A primary advantage of PAL is that the frequency and variety of feedback is increased relative to traditional supervisor–student arrangements due to the many additional opportunities between peers. To support learners' engagement with feedback and evaluative judgement, it is recommended to implement a formal critical reflection framework which is relevant to the learning objectives, activities and levels of learners. Further, this framework should be adjusted as needed to ensure that reflection on the process of learning including peer collaboration is valued as well as the learning activity and outcomes.

Multi-directional peer feedback should include the following.

- **Preparation for peer feedback**: Ensure that learners are prepared for productive peer feedback exchanges from the start. This may require directive guidance in the beginning to ensure that this is constructive and delivered in safe and supportive environment. Learners generally need to develop the skill of engaging in feedback conversations.

- **Clear roles and responsibilities**: Ensure that all peers understand their responsibilities, recognise role limits and know how to seek help when needed.
- **Continuous peer feedback**: Foster ongoing reflection on performance and help learners self-assess and assess the knowledge and skills of others. Foster opportunities to engage in feedback conversations that more naturally occur in a collaborative learning process.
- **Development of evaluative judgement**: Encourage the development of evaluative judgement skills through ensuring clarity of expectations, encouraging self-assessment against these expectations by drawing on examples and evidence from multiple feedback sources. Senior peers are able to demonstrate expected levels for junior peers.

Educator feedback should include the following.

- **Ongoing and formal feedback**: Practice educators should provide both specific and ongoing informal and formal feedback on individual performance that is typically delivered weekly.
- **Clear identification of feedback and action**: Clearly identify feedback in interactions and prompt appropriate responses, such as adjusting performance or planning next steps with actions.
- **Considerations of technology for feedback delivery**: Use technology platforms to deliver feedback when educators and learners are not co-located.
- **Encouraging student feedback**: Encourage students to share feedback with educators to enhance reflection, evaluative judgement and communication skills.

Assessment and especially summative (final stage) assessment against learning outcomes or competency standards almost always remains the responsibility of supervising registered health professional, despite any PAL or NPM arrangements. Nonetheless, peer feedback (and, when relevant, client and other collegial inputs) should be appropriately valued for their unique perspectives and so as not to undermine the merit of PAL. Each party's responsibilities are made clear at the outset of and throughout the PAL experience, and both the intended learning outcomes and processes are a key reference point in formal one-to-one supervision sessions throughout the experience. To further ensure that PAL is valued, assessments should always account for skills and attributes developed through collaboration, even when formal objectives relate to individual competencies. For example, developing professional behaviours, teamwork, communication and reasoning are among the skills highly relevant to PAL and should be assessed as part of the learners' achievements as an individual as part of any collaboration. The output of the collaboration and the assessment of individual expected and assessed achievements within any collaborative endeavour needs to be detailed at the outset and monitored throughout, including with opportunities for the exchange of feedback to ensure learners are clear about their learning and assessment within a placement.

Post-placement

The post-placement phase should revisit the placement aims and focus on feedback, evaluation, reflection and debriefing. It must include perspectives from learners, educators, colleagues, patients/service users and higher education institutions. Special attention should be given to the intent behind implementing PAL and the insights gained by each stakeholder, considering both their individual experiences and/or their future placements. Educators and learners should reflect on the development of knowledge, skills and attributes – including both profession-specific and transferable work-readiness skills such as teamwork, feedback and supervision. Educators and organisations should evaluate how PAL was supported, what was learnt and how it can inform their daily work. Strengths, challenges and areas for improvement should be discussed to foster honesty and a continuous cycle of quality improvement.

Resources, funding, capacity, hidden costs

PAL addresses placement shortages in allied health professions, offering a cost-effective solution to meet growing demands (Markowski et al., 2021; Reidlinger et al., 2017; Allison and Thompson, 2023; Pope et al., 2023). While it is a valuable learning approach, implementing PAL requires a significant investment of time and resources to tailor the model and create the necessary supporting materials and structure. By embedding collaborative learning opportunities, PAL reduces the need for educators to manage every aspect of multiple placements and learners, fostering a more efficient and effective learning environment. The design principles provided guide the delivery of placements that build capacity and produce positive outcomes for both learners and practice educators.

PRACTICE EXAMPLES

PAL placements and near-peer placement tutorials: Liverpool Hospital, south west Sydney local health district, New South Wales

Liverpool Hospital is a large tertiary hospital that offers a substantial number of occupational therapy placements to students across inpatient and outpatient/

community clinical settings. The volume of placements offered has meant that service has had to build capacity and be creative with ways to support and maximise learning opportunities for students. This has included routinely offering PAL placement within clinical settings where peer learning is supported and nurtured routinely, particularly within paediatric and outpatient clinical settings. In terms of facilitating PAL placements, the staff have developed a pre-placement and placement delivery model that they can replicate and deliver each time. They have created a suite of learning resources that student can work through with peers in a self-directed way and collaborate with each other for support, feedback and problem solving where required. The PAL placements in this setting work best with level 3 or level 4 undergraduate students where the paperwork is standardised and practice educators have clear examples of the domains of learning required to allow for easier assessment of individual student competency when working as a pair in a clinical setting. This clarity of learning outcomes required at each level reduces the cognitive load on the practice educator and allows for managing multiple students at once, allowing for energies to be expended on creating spaces and opportunities for shared learning. In terms of the near-peer learning opportunities, the service routinely runs near-peer tutorials with students within the service. This is where they have junior students paired with senior students who are on like for like clinical placement settings and they pair them in a tutorial situation to develop learning. In this tutorial, the senior student offers clinical skill development opportunities for the junior students in areas such as initial interviews, paper-based case studies, developing communication and information gathering skills. The tutorials are structured with pre-set scenarios whereby the junior students can have a go at practicing interviews with senior students in a triad format and have the opportunity to discuss and develop skill from paper-based case study examples. The senior students are encouraged to share their experience and learning, and provide feedback to the junior students on their skills and reasoning in a safe space. This allows the junior student to gain practice and feedback on clinical skills in a safe space that has no risk to patients, whilst it develops the senior student's skills of evaluative judgement and giving constructive feedback to junior students, helping develop their leadership and feedback skills. Where aptitude is shown by the senior student, this near-peer learning opportunity can then move to the senior students observing junior students in clinical settings with patients. Within this setting, the near-peer tutorial has become an established practice that is perceived as beneficial by practice educators and students alike.

Podiatry peer-assisted learning clinic, Western Isles, Scotland

A PAL podiatry clinic was established in the rural Western Isles of Scotland to provide students with opportunities to participate in placements outside the more urban and central areas of the country. This model was developed to create capacity within a small and geographically dispersed team to host podiatry students effectively. The placement focused on a two-week programme for level 3 undergraduate pre-registration podiatry students.

To support the implementation of this model, practice educators engaged in training and development through National Health Service (NHS) Education for Scotland services, enabling supervisors to upskill and deliver the PAL approach effectively. Planning involved identifying the learning needs of students to design a tailored placement experience. This resulted in a partially integrated PAL placement, whereby students worked in pairs within a designated clinic. The clinic focused on low-risk patients who had been pre-screened and combined collaborative learning opportunities with individual activities to meet each student's specific needs.

The key learning outcomes for the placement included developing students' experience and competence in initial assessment, treatment planning and clinical reasoning. Teamwork was also a central learning objective. During the PAL clinic, students adopted the following structured three-point check approach with their allocated patients.

1.   Reviewing case notes and developing a preliminary plan.
2.   Conducting an initial assessment to inform treatment planning.
3.   Discussing the assessment outcomes and treatment rationale with the supervisor to ensure accuracy and alignment with clinical reasoning.

Learners worked in pairs to complete the assessments, with one student leading the consultation while the other recorded notes. Throughout the process, the students checked in with each other to ensure that all aspects of the assessment were covered, fostering teamwork and collaborative problem solving. After completing the assessment, the pair collaborated to refine their clinical reasoning and management plan before presenting it to the educator for approval. While the clinic was running, the practice educator remained available for consultation but typically undertook other tasks, such as administrative duties. This approach allowed students to work with greater autonomy while still benefiting from supervision and guidance when needed.

Feedback from students on this placement has been overwhelmingly positive. Learners expressed a newfound consideration for working in rural settings in the future. Learners also reported that learning alongside a peer not only enhanced their clinical skills but also had a positive impact on their wellbeing and socialisation – attributes which are particularly valuable in such a remote location.

Overall, the PAL clinic has evolved into a sustainable and preferred placement model for level 3 podiatry students in the Western Isles. It successfully combines high-quality learning experiences with peer support and rural healthcare exposure, offering a valuable and effective approach to student education.

Primary care occupational therapy PAL placement, NHS Grampian, Scotland

Based in a primary care service in rural Scotland, this placement example supported two final-year occupational therapy students to work within a clinical setting to deliver a project-based placement to support quality improvement within the service. The primary care service had been funded on a temporary basis and the PAL student project was focused on gathering service-user evaluation of their experience of the service. The aim of this was to provide evaluation data to provide evidence for securing ongoing funding for the service. The placement was part-time clinical work – including carrying a caseload – and part-time project work; this combined approach allowed students to meet the learning outcomes required of the placement. The practice educator set up the project element of the placement with a clear focus and tangible outcomes that was embedded directly in contributing to the service evaluation and overall improvement plan. This alignment of the student work with a clear focus on contributing to something bigger helped "bind" the students in their collaboration and motivate them to feel part of something important and significant for that service. The practice educator designed the placement with a clear placement timetable and expectations that initially she directed and then gradually handed over to the students as they developed their independence and aptitude with time management and case load management skills. This pre-planning of student time is a central design principle of PAL placements to ensure that learners understand expectations and that collaborative aspects of their placement are clearly outlined and timetabled and are mapped to learning outcomes expected so both students and practice educators have a clear focus and shared understanding. In the first week, a SCOT (strength, challenges, opportunities, and threats) analysis was completed by each learner. This provided a reflective tool to present to the practice educator and each other to allow them to consider their similarities and differences as learners and support them to decide how they best work together and support each other during the placement. This process of how they work together, and their own learning needs, was repeated at halfway to update and revise working arrangements based on progress. The students were encouraged to provide peer feedback and support on a weekly basis, as well as having individual supervision time to review and monitor progress against learning outcomes. This provided the chance for students to develop their appraisal of their own and other abilities and therefore develop evaluative judgement as well as developing skills for giving and receiving feedback with peers, skills required for autonomous graduate practice. Overall, the students completed a successful PAL project placement that delivered on the evaluation of the service-user experience of the service and helped contribute to the ongoing funding of the service. This is something that could not have been easily achieved by the occupational therapists and support staff working on the project due to limited resources.

SUMMING UP

PAL offers a structured, collaborative approach to allied health placements that facilitates learning outcomes, supports placement capacity and fosters essential professional skills such as teamwork, problem solving, professional reasoning and evaluative judgement. The rationale for adopting PAL should be driven by clearly defined learning outcomes and a deliberate design that leverages peer interaction to enrich the placement experience for same-level or near-peer learners. This approach to peer learning has been evidenced to facilitate stress management and health for learners whilst on placement.

While PAL offers a cost-effective strategy to address placement shortages, it also demands time and resources to establish effective frameworks and ensure sustainability. Successful implementation of PAL requires thoughtful planning and preparation, including the selection of supervision models and strategies for peer learning and feedback, with alignment of tasks to the levels and learning goals of students. Practice educators play a pivotal role in creating supportive environments, facilitating learning, monitoring progress and ensuring appropriate feedback and assessment structures are in place. In conclusion, a well-designed PAL placement fosters a culture of collaboration, reflection and continuous improvement – benefiting learners, educators and service users alike.

REFERENCES

Allison, C. and Thompson, K. (2023). Increasing capacity by moving away from one-to-one clinical supervision: Using peer assisted learning and group model of student placements in community paediatric speech and language therapy to enable student-led service delivery. *International Journal of Language and Communication Disorders*, *58*, pp. 2200–2211. https://doi.org/10.1111/1460-6984.12936

Beveridge, J. and Pentland, D. (2020). A mapping review of models of practice education in allied health and social care professions. *British Journal of Occupational Therapy*, *83*(8), pp. 488–513. https://doi.org/10.1177/0308022620904325

Boud, D. (2001). Introduction: Making the move to peer learning. In D. Boud, R. Cohen and J. Sampson (Eds.), *Peer Learning in Higher Education: Learning from and with Each Other* (p. 117). London: Kogan.

Boud, D. and Middleton, H. (2003). Learning from others at work: Communities of practice and informal learning. *Journal of Workplace Learning*, *15*, pp. 194–202. https://doi.org/10.1108/13665620310483895

Brierley, C., Ellis, L. and Reid, E. (2022). Peer-assisted learning in medical education: A systematic review and meta-analysis. *Medical Education in Review*, *56*, pp. 365–373. https://doi.org/10.1111/medu.14672

Briffa, C. and Porter, J. (2013). A systematic review of the collaborative clinical education model to inform speech-language pathology practice. *International Journal of Speech-Language Pathology*, *15*(6), pp. 564–574. https://doi.org/10.3109/17549507.2013.763290.

Callese, T., Strowd, R., Navarro, B., Rosenberg, I., Waasdorp Hurtado, C., Tai, J., et al. (2019). Conversation starter: Advancing the theory of peer-assisted learning. *Teaching and Learning Medicine*, *31*(1), pp. 7–16. https://doi.org/10.1080/10401334.2018.1550855.

Carey, M. C., Kent, B. and Latour, J. M. (2018). Experiences of undergraduate nursing students in peer assisted learning in clinical practice: A qualitative systematic review. *JBI Database of Systematic Reviews and Implementation Reports*, *16*(5), pp. 1190–1219. https://doi.org/10.11124/JBISRIR-2016-003295

Hari, R., Caprez, R., Dolmans, D., Huwendiek, S., Robbiani, S. and Stalmeijer, R. E. (2022). Describing ultrasound skills teaching by near-peer and faculty tutors using cognitive apprenticeship. *Teaching and Learning in Medicine*, *36*(1), pp. 33–42. https://doi.org/10.1080/10401334.2022.2140430

Jassim, T., Carlson, E. and Bengtsson, M. (2022). Preceptors' and nursing students' experiences of using peer learning in primary healthcare settings: A qualitative study. *BMC Nursing*, *21*(66). https://doi.org/10.1186/s12912-022-00844-y

Lave, J. and Wenger, E. (1991). *Situated Practice: Legitimate Peripheral Participation*. Cambridge, UK and New York: Cambridge University Press.

Loda, T., Erschens, R., Loenneker, H., Keifenheim, K. E., Nikendei, C., Junne, F., Zipfel, S. and Herrmann-Werner, A. (2019). Cognitive and social congruence in peer-assisted learning – a scoping review. *PLOS One*, *14*(9), p. e0222224. https://doi.org/10.1371/journal.pone.0222224

Markowski, M., Bower, H. and Essex, R. (2021). Peer learning and collaborative placement models in health care: A systematic review and qualitative synthesis of the literature. *Journal of Clinical Nursing*, *30*(11–12), pp. 1519–1541. https://doi.org/10.1111/jocn.15661

Palsson, Y., Marternsson, G., Swenne, C., Mogensen, E. and Engstrom, M. (2021). First-year nursing students' collaboration using peer learning during clinical practice education: An observational study. *Nursing Education Practice*, *50*. https://doi.org/10.1016/j.nepr.2020.102946

Patton, N., Higgs, J. and Smith, M. (2018). Clinical learning spaces: Crucibles for practice development in physiotherapy clinical education. *Physiotherapy Theory and Practice*, *34*(8), pp. 589–599. https://doi.org/10.1080/09593985.2017.1423144

Penman, M., Tai, J., Evans, G., Brentnall, J. and Judd, B. (2024). Designing near-peer mentoring for work integrated learning outcomes: A systematic review. *BMC Medical Education*, *24*, p. 937. https://doi.org/10.1186/s12909-024-05900-6

Penman, M., Tai, J., Thompson, T. and Thomson, K. (2021). Feedback practices as part of signature pedagogy for clinical placements. *Assessment in Education: Principles, Policy & Practice*, *28*(2), pp. 151–169. https://doi.org/10.1080/0969594X.2021.1892587

Pope, K., Barclay, L., Dixon, K. and Kent, F. (2023). Models of pre-registration student supervision in allied health: A scoping review. *Focus on Health Professional Education*, *24*(2). https://doi.org/10.11157/fohpe.v24i2.559

Reidlinger, D. P., Lawrence, J., Thomas, J. E. and Whelan, K. (2017). Peer-assisted learning and small group teaching to improve practice placement quality and capacity in dietetics. *Nutrition & Dietetics*, *74*(4), pp. 349–356. https://doi.org/10.1111/1747-0080.12293

Secomb, J. (2008). A systematic review of peer teaching and learning in clinical education. *Journal of Clinical Nursing*, *17*(6), pp. 703–716. https://doi.org/10.1111/j.1365-2702.2007.01954.x

Sevenhuysen, S. L., Nickson, W., Farlie, M. K., Raitman, L., Keating, J. L., Molloy, E., Skinner, E., Maloney, S. and Haines, T. P. (2013). The development of a peer assisted learning model for the clinical education of physiotherapy students. *Journal of Peer Learning*, *6*.

Sevenhuysen, S., Thorpe, J., Molloy, E., Keating, J. and Haines, T. (2017). Peer-assisted learning in education of allied health professional students in the clinical setting: A systematic review. *Journal of Allied Health*, *46*(1), pp. 26–35.

Tai, J., Canny, B. J., Haines, T. P. and Molloy, E. K. (2016). The role of peer-assisted learning in building evaluative judgement: Opportunities in clinical medical education. *Advances in Health Sciences Education: Theory and Practice*, 21(3), pp. 659–676.

Tai, J., Penman, M., Chou, C. and Teherani, A. (2021). Learning with and from peers in clinical education. In D. Nestel, G. Reedy, L. McKenna and S. Gough (Eds.), *Clinical Education for the Health Professions Theory and Practice*. Springer.

Vygotsky, L. S. (1978). *Mind in Society: The Development of Higher Psychological Processes*. Cambridge, MA: Harvard University Press.

Wenger, E. (1998). *Communities of Practice: Learning, Meaning, and Identity*. Learning in Doing. Cambridge: Cambridge University Press.

Chapter 5

Long-arm supervision

*Eric Nkansah Opoku, Rosemary Xorlanyo
Doe-Asinyo and Isaac Amanquarnor*

CHAPTER OVERVIEW

Healthcare education is constantly evolving, and the idea of supervising students on placement is changing, too. Long-arm supervision, also known as off-site practice supervision, has emerged as a dynamic model of supervision whereby a supervisor who is located at a distance from the practice placement setting takes responsibility for supervising and supporting the students. This chapter will explore long-arm supervision, clarifying its fundamental design features and exploring its multifaceted implications for allied health education. We will also critically examine the research evidence to clarify the empirical underpinnings of this model. Drawing upon practical case studies, we will present practical applications of long-arm supervision and discuss future directions of the supervision model.

CHAPTER OBJECTIVES

The objectives of this chapter are the following.

- To present an overview of long-arm supervision for allied health education.
- To critically discuss the research evidence on long-arm supervision and the benefits, challenges and approaches to best practice when delivering this model of practice placement supervision.
- To discuss the design features of the long-arm supervision model.
- To utilise real-life case studies as illustrative examples of long-arm supervision.

DOI: 10.4324/9781003411765-5

INTRODUCTION

As healthcare and social care education continues to evolve, supervision remains a fundamental pillar, guiding the growth and competence of aspiring allied health professionals (Knight et al., 2021). The exploration of long-arm supervision as a model of practice supervision challenges conventional notions of what constitutes effective supervision in allied health professions education. Unlike traditional models whereby supervision occurs on-site, long-arm supervision introduces a paradigm shift by leveraging remote technologies to bridge the gap between supervisors and students. This approach is particularly pertinent considering the rapid advancement in technology, the evolving healthcare priorities and the need to modernise educational practices (Knight et al., 2022; Dancza et al., 2013).

In this chapter, we will focus on long-arm supervision, exploring its intricacies, its design features and its benefits and challenges. We will also explore practical implementation of this approach to supervision, drawing insights from real-life case studies and research evidence. To begin our exploration, we will define long-arm supervision and highlight its distinguishing characteristics.

WHAT IS LONG-ARM SUPERVISION?

Traditionally, supervision has been associated with in-person and on-site guidance, whereby supervisors are physically present within the practice setting to offer support and mentorship. Long-arm supervision, sometimes referred to as off-site practice supervision, is a model of supervision whereby a supervisor who is located at a distance to the practice-based learning environment takes responsibility for supervising and supporting the students on placement (Kelly et al., 2023).

As a core principle, supervision responsibilities are allocated to individuals who may not be physically present at the practice site but possess the expertise and knowledge necessary to guide students effectively. While on-site guidance may be provided by staff or practitioners within the service not typically of the same profession, this is complemented by professional guidance from either a university tutor or a practitioner of the same profession (Opoku et al., 2022; Kuusisto et al., 2022; Boniface et al., 2012). Effective collaboration between the long-arm supervisor and on-site practitioners is essential; while the later facilitates hands-on learning experiences, the former offers remote guidance and oversight.

Various strategies and technologies are utilised in long-arm supervision to facilitate effective communication and collaboration between the on-site and off-site supervisors and the students. Virtual platforms – such as video conferencing software and other telecommunication systems – serve as conduits for remote supervision, allowing long-arm supervisors to engage with students in real time and provide timely feedback on their clinical practice. Additionally, asynchronous communication tools – such as email and messaging applications – enable ongoing dialogue and support between supervisors and students, nurturing a sense of continuity and mentorship despite physical distance (Matson et al., 2023).

WHY LONG-ARM SUPERVISION?

The integration of long-arm supervision into practice placements for allied health professions students signifies a strategic response to the evolving nature of healthcare, technology and education. This supervision approach has the potential to mitigate challenges with a shortage of discipline specific supervisors and geographical barriers, ensuring that students in remote or underserved areas have equal access to supervision (Knight et al., 2022; Boniface et al., 2012; Dancza et al., 2013). The potential for the long-arm supervision approach to address these critical challenges was exemplified in Ghana during the early stages of the occupational therapy profession (Opoku et al., 2022). With only two occupational therapy professionals in the country, doubling as university educators, long-arm supervision was used to provide essential guidance and support to students on placement. Long-arm supervision proved invaluable in laying the foundation for the development of the occupational therapy profession in Ghana, enabling students to receive quality supervision and mentorship despite geographical constraints, contributing to the growth and advancement of the profession within the country (Opoku et al., 2022).

The benefits of long-arm supervision extend beyond regions with shortages in allied health professionals. Even in countries and settings where allied health practice is well established, long-arm supervision can play a vital role in enhancing the quality and accessibility of placement experiences. For instance, in role-emerging placements when allied health learners explore non-traditional practice settings and/or pioneer new practice areas, long-arm supervision can play an integral role. By leveraging technology and remote communication, experienced educators and practitioners can offer specialised guidance and support to students across diverse clinical settings. This approach facilitates exposure to a broader range of clinical experiences, promotes collaboration with experts and fosters innovation in practice (Tunprasert and Clarke, 2024; Boniface et al., 2012).

Additionally, long-arm supervision enables students to access supervision from professionals located in different regions or countries, enriching their learning experiences with diverse perspectives and approaches. Thus, regardless of the local context, long-arm supervision stands as a versatile and valuable approach for optimising placement supervision (Opoku et al., 2022).

By eliminating the necessity for physical presence, long-arm supervision optimises the supervision process, minimising travel costs and time constraints for both students and supervisors. Additionally, it ensures consistent support throughout the placement duration, guaranteeing a seamless learning journey and enabling students to receive timely feedback and navigating challenges effectively (Beveridge and Pentland, 2020).

As technology keeps advancing in allied health education and healthcare, long-arm supervision equips students with essential skills for navigating the digitalised healthcare environment and fostering proficiency in remote communication and telehealth technologies (Bacon et al., 2022). This will not only strengthen their digital literacy but also enhance their readiness for future practice settings. Furthermore, the model encourages interdisciplinary collaboration and self-directed learning, empowering students to engage in collaborative problem solving and take charge of their professional growth (Stephens et al., 2024). Box 5.1 provides a summary of the benefits of long-arm supervision.

BOX 5.1   SUMMARY OF BENEFITS OF LONG-ARM SUPERVISION

- Enhanced accessibility to supervision for students in remote or underserved areas.
- Flexible scheduling, accommodating both student and supervisor availability.
- Cost-effective solution, reducing travel expenses and time constraints.
- Continuity of support, ensuring consistent guidance throughout the placement.
- Facilitation of interprofessional collaboration and networking opportunities.
- Promotion of student autonomy and self-directed learning.
- Real-time feedback and troubleshooting, fostering immediate skill development.
- Increased exposure to diverse clinical settings and perspectives.

CHALLENGES WITH LONG-ARM SUPERVISION MODEL

Long-arm supervision comes with its own unique set of challenges. Students under off-site supervision may experience a disconnect between the expectations of their on-site staff and those of their off-site supervisors (Dancza et al., 2013). This disparity can lead to confusion and stress as students grapple with the competing demands and objectives of these two groups. Another challenge is the potential loss of students' strong sense of professional identity (Rodger et al., 2007). In traditional placements, students often look up to close professionals as role models who inspire and guide them in their journey. However, in the long-arm model, the absence of immediate role models at the placement setting can leave students feeling adrift. Furthermore, students may express dissatisfaction with their placement learning experience if they lack a tangible role model at the placement setting (Cleak and Smith, 2017). However, these challenges relating to expectations and role modelling can be mitigated with effective communication, support and mentorship.

Also, technology issues such as accessibility issues, connectivity issues and equipment malfunctions pose significant challenge to long-arm supervision. Limitations in face-to-face interaction can potentially affect rapport and communication, and cause difficulties in comprehensive assessment, due to limited observation opportunities. Moreover, disparities in access to technology and digital literacy skills among students – along with privacy and confidentiality concerns regarding remote communication platforms – pose additional challenges (Beveridge and Pentland, 2020; Bacon et al., 2022). However, by proactively addressing these challenges through strategic planning, effective communication and tailored support, institutions can optimise the long-arm supervision model, ensuring a seamless and enriching learning experience for allied health professional students during their practice placements. Box 5.2 summarises potential challenges with long-arm supervision and suggested ways to address them.

BOX 5.2   CHALLENGES WITH LONG-ARM SUPERVISION, AND SUGGESTED WAYS TO OVERCOME THEM

- **Technological barriers, such as connectivity issues or equipment malfunctions**: To overcome these challenges, institutions can provide technical support and resources, conduct regular equipment checks and offer training sessions to ensure proficiency in using remote communication tools.

- **Lack of face-to-face interaction, potentially affecting rapport and communication**: Strategies to mitigate this challenge include scheduling regular video conferencing sessions, encouraging open communication through instant messaging platforms and potentially organising virtual social events to foster a sense of connection and community.

- **The supervisor may have limited observation opportunities, potentially hindering comprehensive assessment of student performance**: Supplemental strategies such as utilising video recordings of clinical sessions, conducting virtual case presentations and incorporating reflective practice activities can help enhance observation and assessment opportunities.

- **Potential disparities in access to technology and digital literacy skills among students**: Institutions can provide equitable access to technology resources by offering training sessions or online tutorials to enhance digital literacy skills and implementing alternative communication methods to accommodate diverse learning needs.

- **Privacy and confidentiality concerns regarding remote communication platforms**: Addressing these concerns will involve selecting secure communication platforms compliant with privacy regulations, establishing clear guidelines for data protection and confidentiality, and providing training on maintaining privacy and security protocols during remote interactions for both students and supervisors.

- **Difficulty in establishing a sense of belonging and support within the remote learning environment**: Creating virtual communities through virtual group platforms, peer support groups and implementing peer-assisted learning can foster a supportive learning environment. Encouraging regular communication, feedback and collaboration among students and supervisors can also help cultivate a sense of belonging and mutual support.

DESIGN FEATURES OF MODEL OF SUPERVISION

This section will delineate the foundational elements of long-arm supervision to provide valuable guidance to educators, students and institutions considering or implementing this model of placement supervision. Exploring the design features of long-arm supervision model will equip stakeholders with essential guidelines to navigate the complexities of off-site practice supervision in enhancing the educational experience of students.

Overarching goal of long-arm supervision

The overarching goal of long-arm supervision is to provide guidance and support to students placed in practice settings where there are no on-site supervisors within their respective fields. In this case, on-site supervision is assumed by professionals from different disciplines, whilst remote supervision is done by university educators or supervisors within the same profession. This ensures that students receive comprehensive supervision and achieve learning in practice-based settings despite the absence of on-site professionals within their professions.

Aligning learning outcomes with the goals of the specific placement

For a successful practice-based placement, it is crucial to ensure that the placement learning outcomes align with the goals of the specific placement setting. It is important to ensure clear and concise learning outcomes that resonate with the unique demands and expectations of the practice placement setting. This alignment fosters a cohesive framework whereby educational objectives are integrated with the practical realities of the placement, maximising the potential for meaningful learning outcomes. A comprehensive understanding of the learning outcomes by the on-site supervisors, off-site supervisors and students is needed to enhance the efficacy of the placement experience.

Communication tools

Effective communication tools serve as indispensable components of long-arm supervision. These include technological devices and structured protocols for communication.

Technology

In contemporary education, technological advancements have led to more effective communication strategies and approaches. Long-arm supervision leverages tools such as laptops, high-speed internet connectivity and mobile phones (where permissible on site). Virtual sessions, complemented by students demonstrating their learning activities in real time, exemplify the efficacy of integrating technology into the supervision process. The use of technological tools serves as an essential conduit for on-site supervisors, long-arm supervisors, students and university educators to connect to enrich the overall placement experiences of students.

Structured protocols for communication

Long-arm supervision relies heavily on the establishment of structured communication protocols, highlighting the need for proper planning. Determining the frequency, timing and mode of communication is essential. Most institutions and placement providers often opt for weekly off-site supervision sessions lasting approximately an hour. Nevertheless, these protocols may need to be customised to suit the unique and diverse nature of practice-based settings.

To enhance communication, students need to be encouraged to engage with reflective practices to foster deeper learning and to get the most out of the off-site supervision sessions. Encouraging the culture of reflection throughout the supervision process allows for deeper learning as students and supervisors gain invaluable lessons from problem-solving processes. Additionally, effective communication between all stakeholders is essential to overcome the many challenges inherent in non-traditional practice-based settings.

Stakeholder engagement

Each stakeholder plays a crucial role. Effective collaboration, communication and engagement are necessary to successfully implement long-arm supervision. Educational institutions mainly provide guidance, whilst practice settings facilitate practical learning. Educational and practice-based administrators coordinate efforts and ensure resources are allocated in all settings. Local and remote supervisors mentor students, providing guidance and assessing progress. In some practice settings, community partners are involved in enriching students' learning experiences by providing real-world contexts and resources (Knight et al., 2021).

Student assessments

Practice-based placements are considered examinations within the academic framework. It is imperative to establish clarity and transparency in the evaluation process. Students and supervisors – both local and remote – must have a clear understanding of the assessment criteria, procedures and expectations. This involves articulating the evaluation method in a manner that is accessible and comprehensible to all stakeholders. Institutions must adhere to best practices in evaluation to ensure fairness, consistency and reliability.

The evaluation process within practice-based placements is a multifaceted approach, involving several assessment methods to measure students' progress and proficiency. Documentation and record keeping are an essential part of this evaluation process, ensuring a quantitative capture of student's performance. Beyond this, qualitative assessments such as student reflections are pivotal in providing exact insights into the student's learning journey. Through the combination of assessment methods, supervisors can provide comprehensive evaluations that reflect students' competencies and professional growth. The process of evaluation within practice-based placements serves as a foundation of academic rigour and accountability, ensuring that academic standards are upheld while facilitating meaningful student learning experiences.

The importance of stakeholder feedback

In long-arm supervision, feedback serves as a valuable tool for stakeholders to assess the efficacy of the supervision model, providing insights into what is working well and what areas require improvement, and enhancing the overall placement experience for students and supervisors alike. Regular debriefing sessions, surveys and electronic tools such as MS Forms facilitate efficient feedback collection. Additionally, traditional methods such as handwritten notes are also effective. In addition to students and supervisors, feedback should also be solicited from other stakeholders involved in the placement, to ensure diverse perspectives are considered, contributing to a comprehensive understanding of the placement dynamics.

Adaptability of the model

The long-arm supervision model is designed to be flexible and adaptable to a diverse range of practice-based settings. Institutions should recognise that these settings vary in personnel, technology and resources, and that they must plan accordingly. By adjusting supervision methods, this model can be implemented effectively in various settings, whether high-resourced or low-resourced. The adaptability feature of this model of supervision enhances students' achievement of practice-based learning outcomes across a wide range of educational environments.

Availability of resources

The effectiveness of long-arm supervision relies on the availability and allocation of resources such as funding, time and personnel. Adequate funding, sufficient time and skilled personnel are required to allow universities to enhance placement site capacity and utilise experienced supervisors. In this model, universities may recruit and compensate experienced off-site supervisors or establish mutually beneficial arrangements with both academics and practitioners. Off-site supervisors are deployed on a flexible basis to support student practice experiences and to ensure effective student evaluation. This model ensures clear and cooperative benefits for all stakeholders (Knight et al., 2022).

Support and training for stakeholders

Comprehensive support and training are imperative for the successful implementation of long-arm supervision, benefiting students, practice educators (on site or off site) and university placement tutors alike. Students, educators and university placement tutors must undergo thorough training to ensure that all parties are equipped with the necessary skills and knowledge. Essential resources – such as placement assessment report forms, marking rubrics and guidelines for supervision frequency and mode – should be clearly provided.

Continuing professional development (CPD) courses, placement briefings and specialised practice education programmes can integrate long-arm supervision concepts, enhancing the preparedness of educators and students alike. Pre-placement training serves to optimise the learning experience for students, enriching their readiness for the demands of practice-based learning.

Off-site supervisors play a crucial role in supporting practice-based learning and must undergo structured preparation to ensure that they possess the requisite knowledge and skills to fulfil their responsibilities effectively, ensuring they adhere to professional standards set by respective professional bodies (Knight et al., 2021).

Recognising the significance of cultural differences in long-arm supervision, emphasis is placed on cultural preparedness for students embarking on placements. Cultural sensitivity and awareness are essential for navigating diverse practice settings and maximising learning outcomes (Overton et al., 2009).

Supervisors involved in long-arm supervision require ongoing support to excel in their roles. This support includes access to resources, mentorship opportunities and avenues for professional growth to ensure the quality and effectiveness of long-arm supervision practices.

Ethical and legal considerations

Long-arm supervision must uphold professional standards, privacy, confidentiality and cultural sensitivity. Formal legal agreements between educational institutions and practice settings provide clarity on roles, responsibilities and expectations, safeguarding the interests of all parties involved. Institutions must implement risk management strategies – including identification, mitigation and contingency planning – to ensure the safety and wellbeing of students and educators. Long-arm supervision must also account for cultural and diversity factors to ensure inclusivity and respect for all participants' backgrounds and perspectives (Table 5.1).

Table 5.1 Design principles of long-arm supervision placements

Rationale for choice of model of placement	The rationale for adopting the long-arm supervision model in practice placements is rooted in its ability to address key challenges and leverage emerging opportunities in healthcare education. Long-arm supervision represents a strategic response to the changing educational needs, the evolving healthcare system and rapid technological advancements. This model of supervision transcends geographical barriers and offers flexible scheduling, ensuring equitable access to supervision while optimising resource utilisation. Moreover, its cost effectiveness and promotion of digital literacy skills prepare students for the evolving nature of healthcare. Long-arm supervision also fosters interdisciplinary collaboration and self-directed learning, empowering students to thrive in diverse practice settings (Stephens et al., 2024).
Can the placement be supported as PAL?	Peer-assisted learning can complement long-arm supervision by fostering collaboration and peer support among allied health professional students. Peer feedback, shared experiences and collaborative problem solving can enrich the learning process and enhance the effectiveness of long-arm supervision.
Approach to supervision	Long-arm supervision is typically delivered through a combination of video conferencing, telecommunication and online collaboration platforms. Supervisory sessions may involve virtual meetings, asynchronous communication via email or messaging apps and access to online resources and learning materials.
Planning and preparation	Planning for long-arm supervision involves identifying technological requirements, establishing communication protocols, scheduling supervisory sessions and clarifying roles and responsibilities of both students and supervisors.

Table 5.1 continued

	Preparation may also include training on digital tools, setting expectations for performance and feedback, and ensuring data security and confidentiality.
Implementing placement	Implementing long-arm supervision requires effective communication and coordination among stakeholders including educators, clinical supervisors, information technology support staff and students. Clear communication, regular feedback mechanisms, ongoing evaluation and adaptation of the supervisory process, and addressing challenges as they arise are essential to monitor progress, address challenges and optimise the learning experience. This may also include providing technical support, offering training and support for digital literacy, and fostering a culture of collaboration and continuous learning.
Post-placement	Post-placement, continued support and reflection are essential components of long-arm supervision. Opportunities for debriefing, feedback sessions and follow-up discussions enable students to consolidate their learning, reflect on their experiences and identify areas for further development, ultimately contributing to their professional growth and readiness for independent practice.

LONG-ARM SUPERVISION IN OCCUPATIONAL THERAPY EDUCATION IN GHANA: A CASE STUDY

The University of Ghana occupational therapy programme adopted long-arm supervision to address challenges with the lack of occupational therapy practitioners at health settings in the country. The university partnered with local healthcare facilities to identify suitable practice placement opportunities. Two university educators who were the only occupational therapists served as long-arm supervisors (Opoku et al., 2022), whilst other local professionals served as on-site supervisors. This case study exemplifies the implementation of long-arm supervision model in one of the placement sites for third year occupational therapy students, highlighting the preparation, implementation and post-implementation phases of the placement.

Planning and preparation phase: In the initial stages, thorough pre-planning was essential to lay the groundwork for the long-arm supervision placement. In this instance, students were placed at physiotherapy department, as the setting did not have occupational therapy department at the time. Technological requirements, including internet connectivity and video conferencing tools, were evaluated in preparation for remote supervision. Additionally, well-structured training sessions were organised for students and supervisors to orient themselves with placement learning outcomes and expectations, the implementation of long-arm supervision, and assessment methods, ensuring their preparedness for the placement.

Implementation phase: With the groundwork in place, the implementation of the long-arm supervision placement commenced. Occupational therapy students were deployed to the hospital for their placement, with an assigned university educator. Students worked in pairs across different units in the physiotherapy department to facilitate peer-assisted learning. Throughout the placement, students engaged in various activities, including conducting assessments, delivering interventions and collaborating with healthcare teams. While on-site supervisors provided regular supervision, weekly virtual supervision meetings via Skype and regular phone calls were scheduled between students and university educators to review progress, address challenges and provide guidance. Leveraging on digital messaging platforms such as WhatsApp text messaging, students sought input from remote supervisors, ensuring ongoing support and mentorship. Utilising practice placement logbooks, students documented their experiences and reflected on their learning, as evidence to facilitate assessment.

Post-placement phase: Following the implementation of the long-arm supervision placement, a comprehensive evaluation of learning outcomes and impact of the placement was undertaken. Students and supervisors (both local and remote) convened to debrief on students' learning experiences, share insights and identify areas for improvement. Feedback from hospital staff and patients was essential to assess the effectiveness of services provided through the placement, and identify opportunities for continued collaboration and development. Additionally, students made presentations on their placement experiences and some case studies on which they worked to peers and faculty members to consolidate their learning experiences, fostering knowledge sharing and continuous learning.

This case study highlighted the transformative role of long-arm supervision, demonstrating its potential to address geographical barriers and a shortage of profession-specific supervisors. The lessons learnt from the long-arm supervision placement has laid the foundation for further refinement and expansion of the model in occupational therapy education in Ghana.

Interprofessional PAL placements, University Department for Rural Health, Australia

The University Centre for Rural Health, Lismore is a government funded academic hub focused on workforce development in rural areas within northern New South Wales, Australia. It provides service-learning placements where students from different allied health backgrounds – such as occupational therapy, speech and language therapy, physiotherapy nutrition and dietetics, and social work – are placed together in pairs and/or small teams within primary health services, such as schools or residential aged care homes. These rural primary health services tend not to have allied healthcare staff on site, and supervision and support is provided via a long-arm supervision model from educators employed through the university. The students are organised in discipline or interprofessional pairs and tend to be either level 3 or level 4 of their undergraduate programmes or second year within their MSc pre-registration programmes. Therefore, they tend to be students nearing the end of their education and learning outcomes are focused on developing professional identity, interpersonal skills, collaboration and teamwork, discipline specific reasoning and caseload management commensurate with graduate-level practice.

A student-centred approach is taken, whereby educators guide student pairs and/ or interprofessional student teams through key learning objectives in the initial weeks of their placement. This supports students to develop their knowledge of their roles and those of others within a team environment and build their confidence and skills in all aspects of the clinical reasoning cycle. Students are provided with a small caseload from day 1 and are required to work through weekly tasks with their peers. During week 1, students are tasked with defining their role and understanding the roles of other team members. They may spend time shadowing staff and other allied health students within the service. Additionally, week 1 is focused on gathering information and completing initial assessments on their focus clients. Week 2 and week 3 are focused on person-centred goal setting conversations, gathering baseline data and setting short-term intervention objectives. Week 4 is focused on planning for and delivering person-centred interventions that are measurable and aligned to their professional scope of practice. This structured four-week programme allows for placements to either be sped up or slowed down, depending on the students' assessed confidence and skill level with each task. As students increase their level of competency, their caseload increases and they continue working through these objectives.

During the placement, the student is supported to engage in regular supervision with their practice educator. This can be completed in person or via Zoom, tutorials or phone calls, and is student led. The students are encouraged to engage with peer learning whilst working with clients together to develop interprofessional teamwork, problem solving and clinical reasoning skills. They are encouraged to observe each other in clinical settings and provide peer feedback on communication and shared professional skills, ethical practice and values required of a health and social care setting. The students are encouraged to provide daily informal feedback and support to provide a 'sounding board' for each other to share ideas, reasoning and thinking about client needs, goals and interventions. These placements rely on PAL principles of design to provide a shared, safe learning space for students to develop skills and confidence.

CONCLUSION

Long-arm supervision represents a comprehensive framework encompassing essential features such as communication, goals and objectives, stakeholder engagement, student assessments and feedback, adaptability, resources, ethical and legal considerations, and support and training. By integrating these key elements, long-arm supervision offers a holistic approach to education, fostering accessibility, flexibility and excellence in student learning experiences. As the nature of healthcare, health educational and technology continue to evolve, long-arm supervision remains an indispensable tool, providing innovative solutions to emerging challenges and shaping the future of allied health professional education and practice.

REFERENCES

Bacon, R., Hopkins, S., Kellett, J., Millar, C., Smillie, L. and Sutherland, R. (2022). The benefits, challenges and impacts of telehealth student clinical placements for accredited health programs during the COVID-19 pandemic. *Frontiers in Medicine*, *9*, p. 842685.

Beveridge, J. and Pentland, D. (2020). A mapping review of models of practice education in allied health and social care professions. *British Journal of Occupational Therapy*, *83*(8), pp. 488–513.

Boniface, G., Seymour, A., Polglase, T., Lawrie, C. and Clarke, M. (2012). Exploring the nature of peer and academic supervision on a role-emerging placement. *British Journal of Occupational Therapy*, *75*(4), pp. 196–201.

Cleak, H. and Smith, D. (2017). Student satisfaction with models of field placement supervision. In *Supervision in Social Work* (pp. 110–125). Routledge.

Dancza, K., Warren, A., Copley, J., Rodger, S., Moran, M., McKay, E. and Taylor, A. (2013). Learning experiences on role-emerging placements: An exploration from the students' perspective. *Australian Occupational Therapy Journal*, *60*(6), pp. 427–435.

Kelly, S., Stephens, M., Hubbard, L., Le Blanc, C. and Breeze, P. (2023). Long arm approaches to practice supervision for non-medical professions: A scoping review. *The Journal of Practice Teaching and Learning*, *20*(3).

Knight, K. H., Leigh, J. A., Whaley, V., Rabie, G., Matthews, M. and Doyle, K. (2021). The supervisor conundrum. *British Journal of Nursing*, *30*(20).

Knight, K. H., Whaley, V., Bailey-McHale, R., Simpson, A. and Hay, J. (2022). The long-arm approach to placement supervision and assessment. *British journal of nursing*, *31*(4). https://doi.org/10.12968/bjon.2022.31.4.247

Kuusisto, K., Cleak, H., Roulston, A. and Korkiamäki, R. (2022). Learning activities during practice placements: Developing professional competence and social work identity of social work students. *Nordic Social Work Research*, pp. 1–14.

Matson, R., Linforth, J. and Edge, C. (2023). Distance supervision as experienced by occupational therapists in mental health: An interpretative phenomenological study. *British Journal of Occupational Therapy*, *86*(9), pp. 622–629.

Opoku, E.N., Van Niekerk, L. and Khuabi, L.A.J.N. (2022). Exploring the transition from student to health professional by the first cohort of locally trained occupational therapists in Ghana. *Scandinavian Journal of Occupational Therapy*, *29*(1), pp. 46–57.

Overton, A., Clark, M. and Thomas, Y. (2009). *A review of non-traditional occupational therapy practice placement education: A focus on role-emerging and project placements*. College of Occupational Therapists, London, England.

Rodger, S., Thomas, Y., Dickson, D., McBryde, C., Broadbridge, J., Hawkins, R., et al. (2007). Putting students to work: Valuing fieldwork placements as a mechanism for recruitment and shaping the future occupational therapy workforce. *Australian Occupational Therapy Journal*, 54, S94–S97.

Stephens, M., Kelly, S., O'Connor, D. and McRae, S. (2024). Reflections on an interprofessional student placement initiative in care homes. *Nursing Older People*, *36*(1).

Tunprasert, T. and Clarke, C. (2024). Diversifying podiatry placements: The future of podiatry education. *Journal of Foot and Ankle Research*, *17*(2).

Chapter 6

Technology-enabled placements

Jennifer Turnbull, Anita Volkert, Susan Pride and Claudine Wallace

CHAPTER OVERVIEW

This chapter explores the role of technology-enabled placements (TEPs) in healthcare education and training. With the rapid advancement of technology, healthcare educators are increasingly leveraging innovative tools and platforms to enhance learning experiences and prepare future healthcare professionals for the complexities of modern practice. The chapter provides an overview of key technologies utilised in healthcare placements, including virtual reality, telemedicine, mobile health applications, wearable devices, data analytics and AI. It discusses the considerations, student expectations and design principles associated with TEPs, emphasising the importance of authenticity, interactivity, personalisation and collaboration in optimising learning outcomes. Furthermore, the chapter examines the evidence base supporting the effectiveness of TEPs and identifies areas for future research and development. Through critical analysis and practical insights, this chapter aims to inform healthcare educators, practitioners, and policymakers about the potential benefits, challenges and opportunities associated with integrating technology into healthcare placements, enhancing the education and training of the healthcare workforce.

CHAPTER OBJECTIVES

The objectives of this chapter are the following.

- To explore the parameters and evidence of TEPs.
- To consider the benefits and challenges of the delivery of TEP.
- To present case study examples as a vehicle for best practice approaches to the delivery of TEP.
- To provide the key design feature of TEP.

DOI: 10.4324/9781003411765-6

INTRODUCTION

TEPs in healthcare have been subject to increasing interest and research due to their potential to improve learning outcomes and provide more comprehensive training experiences for healthcare professionals.

This chapter sets out to define the parameters of TEPs, and consider the benefits, challenges and best practice approaches to their delivery. It will provide a critical review of the research evidence for this model of placement and the design principles key to success with this placement model. It will explore case study examples of TEPs from a range of allied health professions (therapeutic radiography, occupational therapy and orthoptics). The chapter will conclude with reflection on learning and summarise future directions.

The range of technologies on offer within healthcare contexts is ever expanding, and includes (but is not limited to) virtual reality (VR) and augmented reality (AR), which offer immersive experiences that simulate real-world clinical scenarios. Studies indicate that VR and AR can enhance spatial understanding, procedural skills and situational awareness among healthcare learners (Alzahrani, 2020; Papanastasiou et al., 2019).

Telemedicine and telehealth platforms enable remote clinical consultations, patient monitoring and education. Evidence supports the effectiveness of telemedicine in expanding access to healthcare education, facilitating remote supervision and fostering interprofessional collaboration (Budakoğlu et al., 2021).

Mobile Health (mHealth) applications provide resources for clinical reference, learning modules and patient education. Research suggests that incorporating mHealth apps into clinical placements can improve information access, communication and clinical decision-making skills among learners (Maudsley et al., 2019).

Wearable health technology, such as fitness trackers and biosensors, can provide real-time data on physiological parameters and activity levels. Integrating wearable devices into placements offers opportunities for personalised feedback, self-assessment and monitoring of clinical performance (Papi et al., 2015; Sultan, 2015).

Data analytics and AI algorithms can analyse large datasets to identify patterns, predict outcomes and provide personalised feedback to learners. Evidence supports the potential of AI-driven platforms in tailoring educational content, assessing competency and optimising learning pathways in healthcare placements (Piotrkowicz et al., 2021; Luan et al., 2020).

Remote monitoring technologies enable preceptors and educators to observe and provide feedback on learners' clinical activities from a distance. This approach enhances supervision flexibility, promotes reflective practice and supports continuous professional development (Chilton and McCracken, 2017).

TEP also facilitate interprofessional learning experiences by connecting learners from different healthcare disciplines and geographical locations. Collaborative online platforms, virtual simulations and teleconferencing tools promote teamwork, communication skills and shared decision-making in healthcare practice (Bowen, 2020).

Overall, the evidence suggests that TEPs have the potential to enhance the effectiveness, efficiency and accessibility of healthcare education by providing immersive, interactive and personalised learning experiences for learners across various healthcare professions.

WHAT ARE TECHNOLOGY-ENABLED PLACEMENTS?

TEPs refer to educational experiences in healthcare settings that integrate various technological tools and resources to enhance learning, training and professional development for students and professionals. These placements typically involve the use of technologies such as virtual reality, telemedicine, mobile health applications, wearable devices, data analytics and AI to augment traditional clinical experiences.

In TEPs, learners may engage in simulated clinical scenarios, remote consultations, virtual patient encounters and online learning activities that complement their hands-on experiences in real healthcare settings. These technologies can provide opportunities for skills practice, feedback, assessment and collaboration in a safe and controlled environment.

The goal of TEPs is to optimise learning outcomes, foster competency development and prepare healthcare professionals for the complexities of modern healthcare practice by leveraging innovative technologies and instructional methods.

WHY USE TEP: THE EVIDENCE BASE FOR TEP

TEP can provide many advantages in expanding practice-based learning (PrBL) across the allied health professions. The creation of experience-rich new learning opportunities allows higher education institutes (HEIs) to build additional placement capacity, which fits with the UK's National Health Service (NHS) Long Term Plan (2019a, 2019b) to develop sustainable growth in the allied health workforce. TEP also permits HEIs to create learning opportunities for students from and to rural locations, where typically recruitment and retention of healthcare staff is a worldwide challenge (Abelsen et al., 2020). With 91% of English university students also reporting that they were worried about the post-pandemic cost-of-living crisis (Office for National Statistics, 2023), TEP can help reduce expenditure costs for travel and accommodation to learning sites. Additionally, technology continues to develop healthcare delivery, and TEP increases student clinical competence by exposing them to a virtual healthcare environment which patient's pathways are already integrated in to or will be in the future.

The key UK stakeholders in allied health professionals learning all have a clear drive towards digital learning. The strategic framework for NHS Education for Scotland (NES) (2008) requires a workforce with current technological skills to deliver digitally enabled services, while Higher Education England (HEE) (2021) was expanding its digital learning throughout healthcare, with an aim to develop a new generation of digital leaders to drive a technology transformation in the NHS. The High Education Authority (HEA) (2022) recommends that HEIs should take a proactive stance to flexible learning, with technology-enhanced learning (TEL) taking a significant role, as this provides positive outcomes for students. With increasing emphasis being placed on digital learning and services for clinical staff and patients, it is important that TEP are used to prepare students for future employment.

TEP became much more prevalent due to the outbreak of COVID-19 reducing the ability for many students to attend clinical settings in person. Literature published reviewing TEP provide positive encouragement about the success of this model. One study reported on Vietnamese speech and language students, who held case-based discussions with tele-supervisors and utilised videos and avatars. The results show that student satisfaction was high, and their learning outcomes were met (McAllister et al., 2022). A UK study found that a peer-enhanced e-placement (PEEP) offered a successful online placement for health and social care students, meeting learning outcomes, and was accepted by the student body (Taylor and Salmon, 2021; Taylor et al., 2021). An Australian study investigated placements held in an interprofessional style, with structured case studies and discussion held on Zoom. It found that there was increased collaboration, and that there was a reduction in the barriers typically surrounding rural areas (Barraclough and Pit, 2022). Finally, a UK study of dietetic students attending a virtual placement concluded that a vast range of virtual resources could be utilised. Benefits of this model in comparison to standard PrBL were that it was of minimal risk to students and their patients/clients/service users, and that it allows students to revisit and reflect in a way not possible when working in more traditional health and social care settings (Taylor et al., 2021).

Of course, TEP were not invented during the pandemic, with simulated learning already taking a large place in allied health professional education in many HEIs. For example, it has been reported that simulated learning with the virtual environment in radiotherapy (VERT) results in therapeutic radiography students gaining higher confidence in setup, technique knowledge and understanding of machinery involved (Cheung and Wong, 2022). The design of the TEP is fundamental to its success. As with all educational programmes, learning theory should be built in. Figure 6.1 outlines the steps to undertake to develop an effective TEP. Effective feedback is also critical to any learning experience, and this must be considered carefully in the design of TEP. Figure 6.2 outlines key questions to be asked about feedback.

MANAGING STUDENT EXPECTATIONS ON TEP

Practice-based learning environment requirements are documented by professional standards and regulations (Health and Care Professions Council, 2017; NES Education for Scotland, 2008). Research shows that allied health professional students are more engaged in their education when working

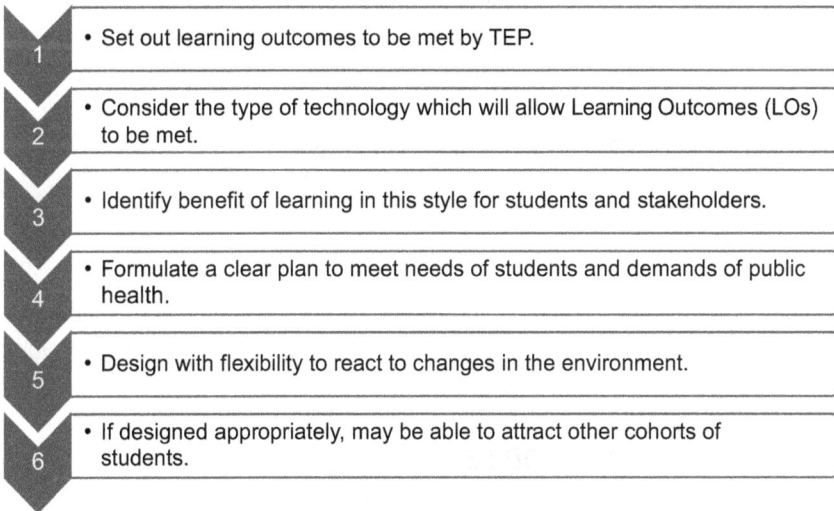

1 • Set out learning outcomes to be met by TEP.

2 • Consider the type of technology which will allow Learning Outcomes (LOs) to be met.

3 • Identify benefit of learning in this style for students and stakeholders.

4 • Formulate a clear plan to meet needs of students and demands of public health.

5 • Design with flexibility to react to changes in the environment.

6 • If designed appropriately, may be able to attract other cohorts of students.

Figure 6.1 Steps in design of successful TEP.

Learning outcomes (LOs)

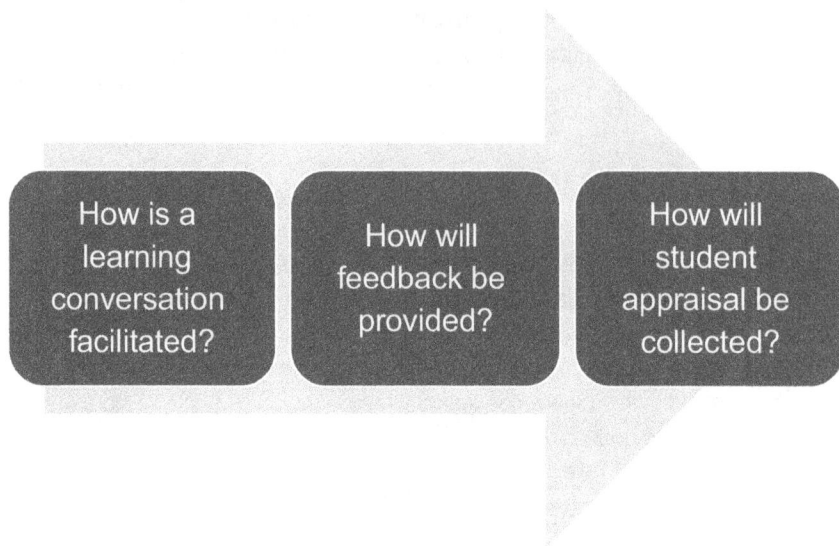

Figure 6.2 Questions to ask about feedback provision and collection

within learning environments and with practice educators who fulfil their needs. It is therefore important to consider what allied health professional students value and consider how to adapt this when designing and implementing a TEP experience. A systematic review reported that allied health professional students value educators who provide effective feedback, foster collaborative learning, understand expectations and have excellent teaching skills (Gibson et al., 2019). Additionally, the most effective learning occurs when students feel comfortable in their learning environment, supported and integrated into the team, and their experiences are professionally managed and organised. Unrealistic expectations of practice-based learning play a significant role in course attrition (McAnulla et al., 2020). It is imperative to manage student expectation and provide clear communication around the design of technology-enabled learning.

Figure 6.3 details some common pitfalls identified in allied health professional online placements (Rossiter et al., 2023) and provides suggestions on how to avoid potential problems with student engagement.

DESIGN PRINCIPLES OF TEP

The design of TEPs in healthcare should incorporate several key features to maximise their effectiveness and relevance to learners' educational needs. Essential design features include (but are not limited to) the following.

Role modelling

- Involve clinical experts in development of TEL from early stage.
- Consider how professional skills and values will be communicated.

Reliance on technology

- Create a "who will contact" guide in case of IT issues.
- Create clear "how to" instructional demo videos.
- Ensure there is technology accessible for students to "loan".

Learning environment

- Create guidelines on appropriate places to learn.
- Develop clear learning outcomes.
- Transparent support method available to the student.

Feedback methods

- Explain to the students the method in which feedback will be provided.
- Verbal and written feedback can successfully be utilised with many TEL.
- Students may find short multiple choice quizzes useful to assess their learning.

Accessibility

- Consider user interface design.
- Assess on a case-by-case basis.

Collaboration

- Consider methods to incorporate peer discussion, with focused questions.
- Design a project to be completed as a group.

Figure 6.3 Common pitfalls identified in allied health professional online placements

Integration of technology: TEPs should seamlessly integrate various technological tools and resources – such as simulation software, virtual reality environments, telemedicine platforms and mobile health applications – into the learning experience. The selection of technology should align with the learning objectives and be placed in or simulate the relevant real-world clinical context effectively.

Authenticity and realism: The placement design should strive to offer authentic clinical experiences that are situated in or that closely resemble actual healthcare settings. This includes working with real service users or with realistic patient simulations, lifelike scenarios, authentic patient data and accurate clinical environments to enhance learners' immersion and engagement.

Interactivity and engagement: Interactive elements should be incorporated to promote active engagement and participation among learners. This may include opportunities for hands-on practice in real or simulated situations, decision-making tasks, role-playing exercises and interactive feedback mechanisms to enhance learning retention and motivation.

Personalisation and adaptability: The placement design should be adaptable to learners' individual needs, preferences and skill levels. Personalised learning pathways, adaptive feedback and tailored educational content can enhance learners' autonomy and address their specific learning goals and challenges.

Feedback and assessment: Robust feedback mechanisms should be integrated to provide learners with timely and constructive feedback on their performance. This may include feedback from instructors, peers, service users and simulated patients, as well as automated feedback generated by technology-driven assessment tools and algorithms.

Collaboration and teamwork: Opportunities for interprofessional collaboration and teamwork should be facilitated within TEPs. Learners from different healthcare disciplines can collaborate on real or simulated cases, participate in team-based activities and practice communication skills to promote effective teamwork and patient-centred care.

Flexibility and accessibility: The placement design should be flexible and accessible to accommodate diverse learning needs, schedules and preferences. This may involve offering both synchronous and asynchronous learning activities, providing remote access to resources and ensuring compatibility with different devices and platforms.

Ethical and professional considerations: Ethical and professional considerations should be integrated into the design of TEPs to ensure that learners adhere to professional standards, ethical guidelines and patient confidentiality. This includes addressing issues such as informed consent, privacy protection and ethical decision-making in both real and simulated scenarios.

By incorporating these key design features (Table 6.1), TEPs can provide learners with rich, immersive and effective educational experiences that prepare them for the complexities of modern healthcare practice.

CASE STUDY EXAMPLES

Therapeutic radiotherapy TEP case study

Professional requirement for TEP

PrBL in therapeutic radiography can be divided into two broad themes: pre-treatment and treatment. Radiotherapy treatment planning is a crucial aspect of pre-treatment, taking place after the patients' scan and prior to treatment. Computer systems precisely locate and calculate dose to the cancer. However, traditional placements are difficult to obtain, resulting in an irregular experience

Table 6.1 Design principles of TEP

Rationale for choice of model of placement	To achieve authenticity, situations where technology is already in use as part of an allied health professional role – or the potential for its use – is being considered. Additionally, TEP work well as part of research, project, long-arm/distance – rural and remote – placements, particularly where there is already a focus on technology (e.g., in a research or project placement). As with any placement decision, the rationale should be clearly thought out in advance and communicated to students and relevant stakeholders.
Can the placement be supported as PAL?	Yes, TEP lend themselves well to PAL approaches as can be seen in the previously discussed design principles.
Approach to supervision	Supervision may be remote (long-arm) or face to face. Supervision within allied health professional placements is usually offered in a formal capacity weekly, with additional and informal supervision and support on an ad hoc basis. Formal supervision always benefits from being planned, regular, documented and using a model to guide content and discussion (Dancza et al., 2023). Placement assessment within allied health professions is usually continuous, with halfway and final assessments. In some situations, these can be formative, or non–credit-bearing, and in others they are summative and credit-bearing.
Mode of delivery	Varying – TEP can be remote, partially remote or in person, depending on the type of technology being utilised. This will depend on the practice context and the aims and goals of the specific placement.
Planning and preparation	In advance, consider the types of technology that will be utilised and the rationale. Consider the structure and timetable of the placement – location(s), activities on different days of the week or blocks of time, real vs. simulated, etc. Communicate with students and relevant stakeholders in advance: a preparatory meeting to discuss and document everyone's goals and desired outcomes for the placement is a clever idea, as well identifying relevant development needs.
Implementing placement	Allow time for induction and address development needs specific to the technology early in the placement process. Supervision and regular check-ins should include time to troubleshoot issues with the technology and its use in the placement context. Activity recording methods such as the activity diary (see Appendix 6.1) may help students and practice educators understand, reflect on and appreciate the relationship between placement activities and learning.

Table 6.1 continued

Post-placement	Allow time for both discursive and, if appropriate, more formal evaluation of the placement experience, as well as the achievement of goals and outcome. Students and stakeholders should reflect on the placement and plan for the next experience, based on learning.

across the student body. The cost of a planning system is prohibitively expensive, so being involved in the development of Varian's Academic Hub, a system shared between HEIs, presented an excellent opportunity to develop a TEP.

Delivery methods

The Hub is a cloud-based resource permitting simulated treatment planning with the latest technologies. Learners can access the placement from any computer, allowing flexibility in teaching delivery methods. Delivery models have varied: a completely online model was used during the COVID-19 pandemic, while the current approach utilises small tutorials on campuses. Both lecturers and clinical specialists deliver the PrBL, with a different case study explored for each session. Additionally, asynchronous learning packages allow for individual learning at times convenient for the learner.

Experience

The Hub allows for the creation of specific learning packages to meet learning outcomes, ensuring an equitable learning experience and successfully bridging the gap between clinical and academic knowledge. This is turn boosts the student confidence and skills to accurately create effective plans, which result in safe treatment for the patient. Using simulated patients further reduces risk to patients.

Student feedback has demonstrated incredibly positive experiences, with clear links to the relevance of the placement, enjoyment of the practical aspect and strong connections made between academic and clinical practice.

Occupational therapy TEP case study

Between August and October 2020, NHS Lanarkshire hosted a fully online placement. The placement host was the occupational therapy team, and the setting was the stroke and neurology rehabilitation team in North Lanarkshire. The placement was set up in conjunction with Glasgow Caledonian University (GCU), with a final-year occupational therapy student.

Several people were key to the setting up of the placement – information governance, information technology, the local practice education group, the professional lead for occupational therapy and the AHP director – to ensure all the correct guidance was being followed. The student taking part in the placement was able to have access to an NHS laptop, login and email address. The main platform used during the placement was NHS Near Me (a localised version of the Attend Anywhere system); this was used for communicating with the student and for patient contact, as well.

A significant amount of planning took place for this placement, since this was a new experience for all involved. As part of the agreed placement hours, the student had a preparatory week to familiarise herself with the information technology systems and pre-placement reading, alongside some online meetings with the educator. Regular times for meetings were set up during this time, including weekly formal supervision and dates for the halfway and final reports. This protected time allowed for discussions about the day ahead and the opportunity to debrief at the end of the day. It was also important to plan regular conversation time into each day, due to the usual social norms of the placement being removed with it being online.

On days that the educator was screening new patients for the team, student input was especially important and exposed her to the importance of the priority system used for patient referrals. The student was able to be part of home assessments to patient's houses via the educator's mobile phone, whereby she was dialled in via NHS Near Me, and as her confidence grew over the duration of the placement, she was an asset to the assessment process. Many patients were happy to provide their consent for this unusual way of interacting with a student, and most of the patients seen developed particularly good therapeutic relationships with the student. This setup enabled the student to fully consider the occupational therapy process for each individual patient as she observed what the educator observed. Between visits, the time was used constructively in the car to discuss the visit and make plans for further treatment and assessment. When the educator returned to base, most of the patient notes had already been completed by the student and these were then checked and countersigned by the educator.

The team support for the placement was excellent and the student got to know the other members of the team and spent time with them on separate occasions, often seeing the same patient to allow observation of how different professions work whilst considering the occupational therapy position. Through reflection and discussion, the educator was able to assess how well the student was progressing, aided as well by a detailed activity diary (please refer to Appendix 6.1 for a sample copy of the activity diary) kept by the student to monitor her time and what kind of learning she had the opportunity to participate in. The activity diary was evidence that a sizeable number of different opportunities were available to the student that she was able to access just as well as if she had been present at the placement site. The university provided excellent support throughout, particularly with completion of the halfway and final reports. This was an area the educator did find daunting, given how far removed the placement setup was from the norm. It was important to ensure that both the educator and the student provided a detailed account of the placement as evidence that all the learning outcomes were sufficiently met.

This placement was successful from the perspective of both the educator and the student, as well as the wider occupational therapy service in Lanarkshire, and led to the development of further fully online placements. It demonstrated that by harnessing the determination of staff in NHS Lanarkshire and GCU to provide a unique placement experience whilst using the developing technology that we had to welcome during the pandemic, the opportunity for different learning experiences could be embraced by many more occupational therapists.

Orthoptics TEP case study

Following a successful bid to the HEE Clinical Placement Expansion Fund, the British and Irish Orthoptic Society (BIOS) was awarded funds to grow clinical placement expansion. Part of the funding was used to purchase Hololens2 devices for some orthoptic departments. These are cameras worn on the head by the orthoptist whilst assessing patients. The sites have had to follow a rigorous approval process with their NHS boards and trusts to enable their participation in this initiative. Lancashire Teaching Hospitals NHS Trust in the UK was set up in September 2022 with consultations live streamed to students studying orthoptics at the University of Sheffield, University of Liverpool and GCU.

These clinics run every Monday morning. The experienced orthoptist has three patients booked per clinic, and the patient has a one-hour appointment. At GCU the live streaming is attended by third- and fourth-year orthoptic students. The benefits of these sessions have continued well after the university and clinical placements returned to normal following the pandemic. Having meaningful conversations about each case with the lecturer facilitates deeper understanding across a cohort of students and ensures standardisation in practice-based learning.

Initial responses from students are promising. The clinical expansion group presented early data at the International Orthoptic Conference (2022), which showed that students reported improved theoretical and clinical knowledge due to the live stream and recorded patient episodes.

CONCLUSION: KEY PRINCIPLES AND CRITICAL COMMENTARY

We now live and work within a post-pandemic world, and the digital interface and progress made within that time was unprecedented, particularly within the field of healthcare. This progress will continue, and as McComiskie (2023) explained, allied health profession graduates are entering a healthcare system in which digital is part of the answer to every question – and as such, allied health professionals must not be left behind. We must prepare our students for the future practice landscape.

It is therefore imperative that allied health professional students are introduced to digital skills and developments within the practice placement environment, offering them skills to build upon to ensure a basic level of digital competence and confidence once qualified and entering the workforce. This ensures we are providing opportunities for students to embrace digital skills within their future practice.

TEP are not just digital placements but also fitting students out for future practice. As we are now increasingly seeing the advent of digital leads in healthcare, we can hope for further focus and support on TEP moving forward, to embrace the changing face of practice

TEPs in healthcare thus offer promising opportunities to enhance learning outcomes and prepare healthcare professionals for the demands of modern practice. However, a critical commentary also highlights several considerations and potential limitations associated with these placements, which include (but are not limited to) the following (Jones et al., 2022).

Cost and resource intensiveness: Implementing TEPs often requires significant financial investment in equipment, software, infrastructure and faculty training. Additionally, maintaining and updating technological resources can incur ongoing costs. Limited financial resources may restrict access to TEPs for some institutions or learners.

Validity and transferability of learning: While TEPs can simulate realistic clinical scenarios, questions remain about the validity and transferability of learning outcomes to real-world practice. Learners may struggle to apply skills and knowledge gained in simulated environments to diverse clinical contexts, potentially limiting the effectiveness of these placements in preparing them for actual patient care.

Technological barriers and access disparities: Technological barriers such as limited internet connectivity, device compatibility issues and digital literacy gaps can hinder access to TEPs, particularly for learners from underserved or resource-limited settings. Addressing these disparities is crucial to ensure equitable access to educational opportunities.

Ethical and professional challenges: TEPs raise ethical concerns related to patient privacy, confidentiality, and informed consent, particularly in simulated environments where patient data and scenarios are used. Ensuring adherence to ethical guidelines and professional standards is essential to maintain the integrity and trustworthiness of these placements.

Overemphasis on technological solutions: There is a risk of overemphasising technological solutions without adequately considering their pedagogical value or alignment with learning objectives. Effective integration of technology requires careful consideration of instructional design principles, learning theories and educational best practices to ensure that technology enhances rather than detracts from the learning experience.

Lack of standardisation and quality assurance: The variability in the design, implementation and evaluation of TEPs can lead to inconsistencies in educational quality and outcomes. Establishing standardised guidelines, quality assurance mechanisms and accreditation standards for TEPs is essential to ensure educational rigour and accountability.

Human factors and interpersonal skills development: While technology can simulate clinical tasks and procedures, it may not fully replicate the human factors and interpersonal aspects of healthcare practice, such as communication skills, empathy and teamwork. Balancing the use of technology with opportunities for human interaction and relationship building is critical for comprehensive professional development.

Research gaps and evidence base: Despite growing interest, the empirical evidence supporting the effectiveness of TEPs in healthcare education remains limited. More rigorous research is needed to evaluate the impact of these placements on learning outcomes, clinical competence, patient outcomes, and healthcare delivery.

In conclusion, while TEPs hold considerable promise for enhancing healthcare education, addressing the considerations and limitations is essential to realise their full potential and ensure their effectiveness, accessibility and ethical integrity.

THREE TOP TIPS FOR IMPLEMENTING TEP

1. Where technology is used for an aspect of an allied health professional role, consider how this technology can be utilised to provide placements.
2. Explore opportunities to develop student-focused resources with product manufacturers.
3. Develop the PrBL package alongside an expert in the relevant field of technology.

REFERENCES

Abelsen, B., Strasser, R., Heaney, D., et al. (2020). Plan, recruit, retain: A framework for local healthcare organizations to achieve a stable remote rural workforce. *Human Resources for Health*, *18*(63). https://doi.org/10.1186/s12960-020-00502-x

Alzahrani, N. M. (2020). Augmented reality: A systematic review of its benefits and challenges in e-learning contexts. *Applied Sciences*, *10*(16), p. 5660.

Barraclough, F. and Pit, S. (2022). Online multidisciplinary integrated rural healthcare education programs during the COVID-19 pandemic for students from different universities: Experiences and guidelines. *Health Education (Bradford, West Yorkshire, England)*, *122*(2), pp. 202–216. Web.

Bowen, T. (2020). Work-integrated learning placements and remote working: Experiential learning online. *International Journal of Work-Integrated Learning*, *21*(4), pp. 377–386.

Budakoğlu, I. İ., Sayılır, M. Ü., Kıyak, Y. S., Coşkun, Ö. and Kula, S. (2021). Telemedicine curriculum in undergraduate medical education: A systematic search and review. *Health and Technology*, *11*(4), pp. 773–781.

Cheung, E.Y.W. and Wong, C.W.Y. (2022, July). VERT in RT. *Annals of Oncology*, *33*(Supplement 6), p. S521.

Chilton, H. and McCracken, W. (2017). New technology, changing pedagogies? Exploring the concept of remote teaching placement supervision. *Higher Education Pedagogies*, *2*(1), pp. 116–130.

Danzca, K., Volkert, A. and Tempest, S. (2023). *Supervision for Occupational Therapy: Practical Guidance for Supervisors and Supervisees*. Abingdon, Oxon: Routledge.

Gibson, S.J., Porter, J., Anderson, A., Bryce, A., Dart, J., Kellow, N., Meiklejohn, S., Volders, E., Young, A. and Palermo, C. (2019). Clinical educators' skills and qualities in allied health: A systematic review. *Medical Education*, *53*(5), pp. 432–442.

HEA. (2022). *HEA Flexible learning: A literature review 2016–2021*. Available at: https://www.advance-he.ac.uk/knowledge-hub/flexible-learning-literature-review-2016-2021

Health and Care Professions Council. (2017). *Standards of education and training*. Health and Care Professions Council. Available at: http://www.hpc-uk.org/assets/documents/10000BCF46345Educ-Train-SOPA5_v2.pdf

HEE. (2021). *HEE review of the year 2020–2021*. Available at: https://www.hee.nhs.uk/sites/default/files/HEE%20Review%20of%20the%20Year%20-%202020-21.pdf

Jones, A., Wilson, I., McClean, S., Kerr, D. and Breen, C. (2022). Supporting the learning experience of health-related profession students during clinical placements with technology: A systematic review. *Review of Education*, *10*(2), p. e3364.

Luan, H., Geczy, P., Lai, H., Gobert, J., Yang, S. J., Ogata, H., Baltes, J., Guerra, R., Li, P. and Tsai, C. C. (2020). Challenges and future directions of big data and artificial intelligence in education. *Frontiers in Psychology*, *11*, p. 580820.

Maudsley, G., Taylor, D., Allam, O., Garner, J., Calinici, T. and Linkman, K. (2019). A Best Evidence Medical Education (BEME) systematic review of: What works best for health professions students using mobile (hand-held) devices for educational support on clinical placements? BEME Guide No. 52. *Medical Teacher*, *41*(2), pp. 125–140.

McAllister, L.L., Atherton, M., Winkworth, A., Wells, S., Le, D.K., Sandweg, K., Nguyen, T.T.T., Henderson-Faranda, N. and Broadmore, S. (2022). A descriptive case report of telesupervision and online case-based learning for speech and language therapy students in Vietnam during the COVID-19 pandemic. *South African Journal of Communication Disorders*, *69*(2), pp. e1–e6. Web.

McAnulla, S. J., Ball, S. E. and Knapp, K. M. (2020). Understanding student radiographer attrition: Risk factors and strategies. *Radiography (London, England, 1995)*, *26*(3), pp. 198–204. Web.

McComskie, E. (2023). *All allied health professionals need a foundation in digital competence*. A blog by @EMAHPInfo AHPscot blog. Available at: https://ahpscot.wordpress.com/2023/09/18/all-allied-health-professionals-need-a-foundation-in-digital-competence-a-blog-by-emahpinfo-euan-mccomiskie/

NES Education for Scotland. (2008). *Quality standard for practice placement*. NHS Education for Scotland. Available at: http://www.nes.scot.nhs.uk/media/323817/qspp_leaflet_2008.pdf

NHS. (2019a). *Long term plan*. Available at: https://www.longtermplan.nhs.uk/publication/nhs-long-term-plan/

NHS. (2019b). *NES strategic framework 2019–2024*. Available at: https://www.nes.scot.nhs.uk/media/kacboen5/nes_strategic_framework_2019_2024.pdf

Office for National Statistics. (2023). *Cost of living and higher education students*. Available at: https://www.ons.gov.uk/peoplepopulationandcommunity/educationandchildcare/bulletins/costoflivingandhighereducationstudentsengland/30januaryto13february2023

Papanastasiou, G., Drigas, A., Skianis, C., Lytras, M. and Papanastasiou, E. (2019). Virtual and augmented reality effects on K-12, higher and tertiary education students' twenty-first century skills. *Virtual Reality*, *23*(4), pp. 425–436.

Papi, E., Osei-Kuffour, D., Chen, Y. M. A. and McGregor, A. H. (2015). Use of wearable technology for performance assessment: A validation study. *Medical Engineering & Physics*, *37*(7), pp. 698–704.

Piotrkowicz, A., Wang, K., Hallam, J. and Dimitrova, V. (2021). Data-driven exploration of engagement with workplace-based assessment in the clinical skills domain. *International Journal of Artificial Intelligence in Education*, *31*(4), pp. 1022–1052.

Rossiter, L., Turk, R., Judd, B., et al. (2023). Preparing allied health students for placement: A contrast of learning modalities for foundational skill development. *BMC Medical Education*, *23*(161). https://doi.org/10.1186/s12909-023-04086-7

Sultan, N. (2015). Reflective thoughts on the potential and challenges of wearable technology for healthcare provision and medical education. *International Journal of Information Management*, *35*(5), pp. 521–526.

Taylor, L. and Salmon, G. (2021). Enhancing peer learning through online placements for health and social care professions. *International Journal of Practice-Based Learning in Health and Social Care*, *9*(2), pp. 1–10. Web.

Taylor, N., Wyres, M., Green, A., Hennessy-Priest, K., Phillips, C., Daymond, E., Love, R., Johnson, R. and Wright, J. (2021). Developing and piloting a simulated placement experience for students. *British Journal of Nursing (Mark Allen Publishing)*, *30*(13), pp. S19–S24. Web.

Appendix 6.1 Resource: activity diary

REPRINTED WITH PERMISSION

For use on all placements but an essential requirement for any placement that is supervised online for all or part of remote TEP placements.

Summary Record of Attendance

Module name and code:	Practice-Based Learning 2 (BSc) (M3B926057)	
Placement dates	From:	To:
Mode of attendance (fully on-site, fully online, or a blend of online and on-site?)		
Placement site/specialty:		

Guidance on how to complete the activity diary can be at the end of this document. Please ensure you have read it in full.

PRACTICE-BASED LEARNING ACTIVITY DIARY

Week 1 beginning (copy template if further weeks are needed)

	Monday	Tuesday	Wednesday	Thursday	Friday	Saturday	Sunday
Morning							
Afternoon							
Evening							
Total daily hours							
Week number:	Total Hours for Week:				Student Signature:		

Activity diary colour coded key

Activity type/colour code (Most pertinent learning outcomes to activity)	Examples of activity
Research activity and CPD (LO 1,2,4,5)	Reading policies and guidelines, researching evidence base, interventions through journal articles, attending tutorials, in-services or online courses, etc.
Supervision (LO 3, 5 – and involves reflection on other LOs)	Formal supervision, reflections halfway and full way report meetings, etc.
Collaboration/Networking (LO 1,2,3,4,5)	Liaising with team members, other services, team meetings, meeting with other students, virtual multidisciplinary team meeting (MDT) shadowing, delegating responsibilities etc.
Assessment/identification of need (LO 1,2,3,4)	Selection and application of appropriate assessment tools and approaches.
Planning & clinical admin (LO 1,2,3,4)	Planning, documentation, report writing, etc.
Intervention (LO 1,2,3,4)	Delivering activities/actions, e.g., individual, group interventions or actions for an organisation rather than patient/client, etc.
Evaluation of service and of service-user interventions/ interactions (LO 1,2,3,5)	Discussion with service users, staff, peers or self-reflection on how assessments or interventions went.
Other	Anything that does not appear to fit in the colour codes should still be recorded without a colour code, e.g., lunch breaks, virtual tea breaks with team.

The following is an example of practice-based learning activity timetable diary (this student had a mix of online and on-site experience).

Week beginning: 15th November

	Monday	Tuesday	Wednesday	Thursday	Friday	Saturday	Sunday
Morning		9–10am Online team meeting 10–12am Researching tele-rehab and local policies	9–9:30am Meeting with supervisor 9:30–11pm Planning online intervention session 11–11:30am Meeting with & learning from speech & language therapist 11:30am–12noon Reviewing intervention plan and making amendments based on greater awareness of communication issues	10–11 Supervision prep: checking LOs, diary and reflections 11–12pm Formal supervision	9–10am Admin, planning next week 10–10:30am Calls to service user but no answers – checking contact details for accuracy and making notes for entry into case notes 10:30–11am Prep for next session 11–12pm Online session with SU		
Afternoon		12–12:30pm Break 12:30pm–2pm Peer meeting to share research 2–2:30pm Call to befriender service 2:30–4:30pm Reading neurology/ anatomy related to patient group	12–12:30pm Break 12:30pm–2pm Joining occupational therapist online for kitchen assessment 2–2:45pm Writing up draft report of kitchen assessment 2:45–3:45pm Reading up on kitchen assessments and patient's condition, to	12–12:30pm Break 12:30–2pm Student meeting to review intervention plans 2:30–3:30pm Observing home visit initial assessment 3:30–4:30pm Writing notes,	12–12:30pm Break 12:30–1pm Case notes 1–2pm Meeting with PE to self-evaluate session 2–3pm Editing case notes 3pm–3.30pm Checking scheduled events for next week and completing department admin is completed.		

	Monday	Tuesday	Wednesday	Thursday	Friday	Saturday	Sunday
			identify other things for report 3:45–4:15pm Meeting with practice educator (PE) to discuss my observations and report 4:15–5pm Refining and completing report for sign off by PE.	identifying goals from assessment 4:30–5pm Call with supervisor to review assessment and goals			
Evening				6:30–8pm Attended 'stroke' support group evening meeting			
Total hours		7.5 hours	8 hours	8 hours	6.5hrs		

Week number:	Total Hours for Week:	Student signature:

Chapter 7

Simulation and placements

Belinda Judd, Jennie Brentnall and Emma Green

CHAPTER OVERVIEW

This chapter addresses the broad topic of simulation-based education and models of placement. Simulation-based education is taken to include approaches that involve immersive learning experiences that replicate aspects of real life to facilitate authentic learning. Acknowledging the broad scope of simulation, this chapter includes considerations relevant to a range of simulation modalities such as mannequins and part-task trainers, role plays with or without moulage or masks, and virtual or augmented reality with or without the use of AI. Unique features of simulation-based education are highlighted, emphasising its learner-centred approach, design tailored to individual learners, equitable experiences and precise control over learning. Theoretical foundations that specifically apply to simulation design, content and debriefing are acknowledged. Considering the vast evidence base for simulation and placements, systematic reviews, randomised controlled trials and influential research and guidelines are highlighted. Design principles supporting simulation as a placement model are outlined, prompting consideration to the model's flexibility and suitability for diverse purposes and promoting attention to the learner level, learning outcomes, resources and desired realism in design decisions. Finally, the chapter concludes with authentic practice examples highlighting the breadth of simulated placements and a concluding summary that offers key messages and future directions.

CHAPTER OBJECTIVES

The objectives of this chapter are the following.

- Outline the scope of simulation and practice placement models.
- Explain how several learning theories are applied in simulations.

DOI: 10.4324/9781003411765-7

- Summarise the high-level evidence and standards that inform simulation design.
- Explore the application of a range of design principles for simulation and placements.
- Provide practical examples applying simulation in allied health.

SIMULATION AND MODELS OF PLACEMENT

Simulation-based education is a broad educational approach in which learners actively participate in immersive experiences that intentionally replicate or elicit aspects of real life to enable authentic learning. Simulation techniques range from role play to mannequin hardware to virtual reality, which can be applied to achieve a level of realism that is suited to learning and engagement for the specific learners and topics. Unlike many placement-based experiences, simulation-based education controls or manipulates aspects of reality for the benefit of the learner rather than learning occurring secondary to service provision. The complexity and features of simulated scenarios and environments can thereby be designed to scaffold learning from beginner to advanced. Simulation may be removed from reality to the extent that only the experience and learning are real within a completely simulated scenario and environment, or it can be used to create specific opportunities to address defined learning outcomes within otherwise real-life scenarios and environments.

Applied to placements, simulation-based education varies according to the level of the learners, learning outcomes, and resources. It is possible to create a holistic and immersive 'placement' learning experience comprised entirely of simulated scenarios in simulated environments (e.g., in a university-based simulation unit). This would include a range of experiences such as session planning, patient/client encounters, documentation, supervision sessions, team meetings, follow-up with other health professionals and handovers between professionals. Alternatively, simulation-based experiences can be used to enable a specific learning objective within another model of placement that provides complementary real-life experience. For example, simulation may be used to provide predictable and repeated practice of a skill before going to see a real patient/client, where suitable patients/clients are not accessible at the relevant time for learning or at a predictable time that can be scheduled for multiple learners and interprofessional teams. The mode of delivery for simulation-based experiences might include face-to-face, online or hybrid approaches as relevant. In all cases, however, simulation will have a degree of immersion and replication of reality that distinguishes it from case study or problem-based learning, paper-based exercises or viewing video recordings. While simulation can be used to assess learning outcomes, this chapter focuses on simulation for learning.

Simulation enables the intentional use of learning strategies such as briefing that anticipates specific learning points that it is known will arise, pauses for just-in-time feedback and instruction, repetition and debriefing to highlight and reinforce learning before reflection. Simulation in placements can complement other experiences to enable a range of authentic learning that may not otherwise be safely attainable at scale or at predictable opportunities (see the design principles section in this chapter for more details). In doing so, simulation can enable equitable, timely, planned and supported opportunities to achieve the following.

- Address scenarios that specifically complement other learning modalities at the time.
- Review performance and receive multi-source feedback, including from simulated participants (e.g., patients).
- Practise with repetition and/or intentional variation to develop and consolidate proficiency.
- Provide predictable and reliable experience of scenarios that are uncommon in real life.
- Support physically and psychologically safe experiences to develop the skills to manage potentially risky situations.
- Enable collaborative learning in interprofessional groups, across distances or when there are other barriers to gathering in person.
- Enhance public safety by ensuring that learners develop and practise their skills in situations when real healthcare outcomes are not at stake.

Simulation can also be used to identify learners who are not yet ready or safe to continue learning in real-life situations, and to create supplemental or remediation opportunities for learners who experience challenges or are underperforming in placements. In these situations, simulation can provide learners with additional exposures to realistic activities and environments without impacting service delivery. Simulation within or in place of other types of placement experiences can thereby protect provider relationships and contribute to the optimal and efficient use of placement capacity for sustainable health professions education at the scale needed for workforce development.

THE UPTAKE OF SIMULATION AND PLACEMENTS

Simulation-based education, with its many applications, forms an integral part of many health professional degree curricula and its incorporation in placement specifically is a rapidly evolving area with a growing evidence base for varied applications (Squires et al., 2022). Simulation as a placement model has been adopted to varying degrees in different countries and allied health disciplines, usually in university-based settings. Simulation within other placement models is more common in conjunction with universities and where simulation centres and staff continuing professional training teams exist but remains underutilised in allied health compared with medicine and nursing.

There are specific barriers to the wider adoption of simulation within or as placements in allied health. These include a lack of familiarity with simulation opportunities and rationales, limited awareness (or conversely, overwhelm by the volume) of the relevant research evidence and how to apply it, few adequately trained staff and apprehension regarding cost and resource allocation. Further, accrediting bodies' acceptance of simulation and its contribution to required placement experiences varies across allied health professions and countries (Royal College of Occupational Therapists, 2019). Akin to any placement model, these obstacles require thoughtful consideration and counterbalance with the anticipated benefits.

The learning theory applications and evidence highlighted in this chapter guide specific design features to facilitate high-quality simulation in placements. Key points from the research evidence and expert experience are also summarised in guidelines and practice standards that promote and enable audits of quality. The growing evidence base also includes design options for resource-constrained environments, enabling simulation to make a real, quality contribution to placement learning.

THEORETICAL FOUNDATIONS OF SIMULATION AS A CLINICAL PLACEMENT MODEL

The theoretical foundations of simulation as a clinical placement model stem from a blend of established learning theories and the unique reflective pedagogy inherent to simulated environments. While various placement models emphasise active student engagement and experiential learning, simulation also places particular emphasis on reflective practice and mastery learning as essential components of its design and application.

In the broader context of learning theories, such as experiential and social learning theories, which are prevalent across most placement models, simulation stands out for its reflective pedagogy. This pedagogy – encapsulated by the notion of "thinking, feeling, and doing" – offers learners a dynamic platform to engage in high-fidelity performance, as noted by Gormley and Murphy (2023). Central to this reflective pedagogy is the theory of mastery learning, originally proposed by Bloom in 1968 (Bloom, 1968). Mastery learning asserts that students must attain a predetermined level of proficiency before advancing to acquire subsequent knowledge and skills. Should a student not meet this mastery criterion during evaluation, they receive additional support tailored to their learning needs. Within the controlled environment of simulation, this theory finds fertile ground for implementation. Here, students benefit from the flexibility and repeated practice afforded by the model, enabling them to progress at their own pace through repeated cycles of learning until mastery is achieved.

EVIDENCE AND STANDARDS

The evidence base for simulation is vast and rapidly expanding, given that simulation is increasingly a critical part of health professional training. This section will therefore focus on systematic reviews, randomised controlled trials of simulated placements in allied health, seminal studies and practice guidelines.

Multiple systematic reviews report positive outcomes of simulation (Alanzi et al., 2017), including in audiology (Alanazi and Nicholson, 2023), nursing (Cant and Cooper, 2010; Hegland et al., 2017), pharmacy (Beshir et al., 2022), physiotherapy (Javaherian et al., 2020; Mori et al., 2015; Pritchard et al., 2016; Rezayi et al., 2022) and social work (Kourgiantakis et al., 2020). There is also good evidence for simulation specifically for interprofessional education (Sezgin and Bektas, 2023; Marion-Martins and Pinho, 2020) and for developing empathy (Chua et al., 2021). Systematic reviews have illustrated the effectiveness of student peers in simulation roles (Dalwood et al., 2020) through to technology-enhanced simulation (Chen et al., 2020; Cook et al., 2011, 2012; Foronda et al., 2020; Kononowicz et al., 2019).

Simulated placements have demonstrated equitable outcomes to more traditional placement models (Bogossian et al., 2019; Larue et al., 2015), with evidence from randomised controlled trials in occupational therapy (Imms et al., 2018), physiotherapy (Watson et al., 2012), radiography (Ketterer et al., 2020) and speech pathology (Hill et al., 2021; MacBean et al., 2013). The consistency of this evidence provides reassurance that student learning outcomes are comparable between traditional and simulated placements, paving the way for greater acceptance of simulated placements and adoption of simulation as a partial replacement or complementary feature within other models of placement.

The application of simulation in placements is founded on a substantial history of thoughtful development that has fostered an emphasis on effective pedagogy, customised design and resource optimisation. Specifically, educators have been implored to use human interaction to develop crucial healthcare skills such as professionalism and communication, expanding simulation beyond the realm of technical task training (Kneebone et al., 2006). Gaba (2004) focused the field's attention on ensuring the relevance and return on investment of simulation-based education through the demonstration of improved patient safety outcomes. Part of this equation is necessarily balancing simulation-based methodologies with other approaches, including real practice experiences (Gaba, 2004). More recently, the imperatives of establishing a psychologically safe learning environment and debriefing with skilled facilitation have broadened attention beyond technologies and to the whole educational approach to simulation.

To inform simulation design, there is international agreement on good practice (Diaz-Navarro et al., 2024), providing priorities for the broad adoption of exemplary simulation practice that benefits patients and healthcare workforces globally. Other organisations have developed best practice guidelines that enable the advancement of simulation, share best practices and provide an evidence-based framework for the practice and development of a comprehensive standard of practice (Diaz-Navarro et al., 2024; Watts et al., 2021; Motola et al., 2013). Standards for simulation-based education play a critical role in promoting quality, consistency, safety, research and professional development within the field. They also contribute to the effectiveness and credibility of simulation as a valuable educational tool across various domains including practice placements, and as such, are a useful practical resource.

Research now extensively supports the effectiveness of simulations in various educational contexts including as a placement model. It often outperforms other learning strategies and has gained broad acceptance across professions. Moving forward, goals now of future research in this area could be to examine the role that simulation design characteristics as a variable play in attaining learning outcomes, learning transfer, duration of effect and translational impacts.

CONSTRUCTION OF SIMULATED PLACEMENTS

As illustrated in Figure 7.1, the design of the simulation activities should balance *uncertainty* and *realism* according to the *level of learner* and *learning outcomes*, and considering the available *resources* and *space and equipment*. Features of the patient/client scenario, environmental setup, setting and extraneous factors can be employed to varying degrees to manipulate and control uncertainty and realism in the simulation activities. For example, the *patient/client scenario* can vary

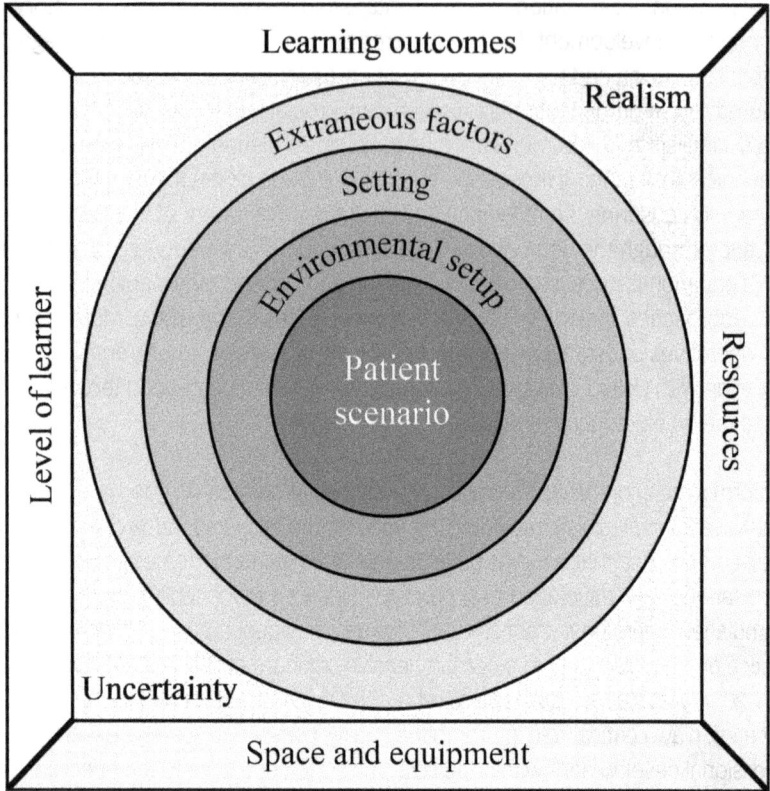

Figure 7.1 The building blocks of simulated placements

in terms of illness and disability features and familiarity, scenario acuity or stability, influencing intrapersonal and interpersonal factors, social determinants, and so on. The mode of delivery and modality of simulation discussed below will contribute to the scenario, augmented by additional information and influences determining the progress of the experience. The *environmental setup* can vary in the level of cues and distractions, offer or withhold resources, and evoke more or less of a response through similarity with the 'real world'. This might include the provision of relevant objects, signage and equipment, or the availability of static or dynamic information about the patient/client status. The human environment is frequently particularly important to learning, including the roles of educators, significant others or carers, other healthcare professionals or ancillary staff, as relevant to the situation. The *setting*, whether it be a hospital, clinic, home or community location, can be established through a simple narrative and imagination or be comprised of a highly realistic replica or even real setting. Finally, *extraneous factors* include any other aspects affecting learning such as distractors that may be present in the scenario, environment or setting, or features of the learners or instructors including physiological and psychological states. These might include irrelevant or conflicting information, noise or phone calls, extended learning sessions or time pressures, and may be desirable where they contribute to realism if they are suited to the level of learners and learning outcomes.

DESIGN PRINCIPLES

Table 7.1 presents a summary of design principles for simulation as a placement model. Key points are summarised in the table, with each design principle expanded on in following text.

Table 7.1 Design principles for simulation as a placement model

Design principles	Key points
Rationale for choice of model of placement	• For novice learners of foundational skills. • For remediation of underperforming students. • For late-stage learners for challenging scenarios or towards work readiness. • To allow controlled opportunities to encounter appropriate levels of complexity and challenge. • To provide consistency of exposure for students. • To provide opportunities for repeated practice of uncommon or sensitive scenarios.
Role of PAL	• The potential to tailor design, control scheduling and offer repetition provides great opportunities for PAL, including in multidisciplinary teams reflecting real practice. • The application of PAL assists learners to maximise the opportunities for repeated practice and peer feedback, and to challenge themselves whilst in a supportive, learner-centred environment.
Role of supervision	• Learner-focused. • Typically facilitative and longer-arm supervision due to less risk to patients and student-led scenarios.
Mode of delivery	• Flexible modes: face to face, online or hybrid. • Modalities include simulated patients, mannequins, part-task trainers, haptic systems, virtual reality (VR), augmented reality (AR) and artificial intelligence (AI).

Table 7.1 continued

Design principles	Key points
Planning and preparation	• Preparing students *how* to learn in simulation. • Training educators how to facilitate in simulation. • Training of actors/volunteers/patients in role portrayal and representation of conditions and scenarios. • Training of other faculty, staff, technicians, etc.
Implementing placement	• Typically follows a cycle of preparation, pre-briefing, simulation activity, debriefing/feedback, reflection and evaluation. • Utilises specific techniques such as pause, rewind and timeouts.
Learner diversity, equity and inclusion	• Provides a controlled and learner-centred environment to cater to a wide range of specific learner needs. • Enables equity of learning opportunities (including catering to different mastery trajectories) whilst replicating aspects of real-life practice placements.
Learner feedback and assessment	• Broad feedback opportunities including from educators, peers, self, simulated patients/participants, other faculty and from AI, VR and AR platforms. • Group debriefing can make sense of and consolidate the learnings. • May create tension between maintaining a safe container of learning in the presence of high-stakes assessment.
Post-placement evaluation and follow-up	• Requires closing the loop with stakeholders (students, volunteers, facilitators, actors, etc.). • Offer support to simulated patients, students and staff to manage emotional load. • Undertake continuous improvement cycles to maximise the opportunities to control and adapt learning instances.
Resources, funding, capacity and hidden costs	• Many considerations contribute to effective and efficient placement model decisions, sustainability, feasibility and capacity building.

Rationale for choice of model of placement

Simulation should be chosen and designed with the level of learner and intended learning outcomes in mind. It is a well-justified approach for placements where it is designed to utilise opportunities to achieve the following.

- Take a learner-centred approach.
- Manipulate and control aspects of the experience.
- Provide scalable learning opportunities at planned and optimal times.
- Incorporate deliberate learning strategies (see also the role of supervision, in what follows) such as briefing, pauses for feedback and instruction, repetition and debriefing.

The ability to design simulation to learners' needs makes it a diversely applicable approach. For example, to provide foundational learning experiences *for novice students*, complexity will be limited to match the students' skill, with realism only sufficient to prompt transfer of learning to real-life settings. To build mastery and confidence, including *for the remediation of underperformance*, uncertainty and realism may be graded over time until (re-)exposure to the real environment is supported. To improve the work readiness of *late-stage learners*, greater degrees of uncertainty and realism provide appropriate challenge and support transferability. *To augment or replace placements* at a planned time that is optimal for learning or to provide exposure to uncommon or sensitive scenarios may require a higher emphasis on realism with uncertainty adjusted to match the intended learning outcomes. In all cases, the learner-centred nature of simulation enables learning by prioritising physical and psychological safety, and support such as through feedback and instruction.

The role of PAL in this model

Simulation is well suited to supporting PAL, given it is learner-centred and limits the impacts on patients/clients and services, including arising from multiple learners participating together. PAL is also ideal to apply to enhance simulation by promoting skill development, increased understanding and knowledge retention, and peer support. PAL assists learners to succeed in complex simulation scenarios requiring teamwork and collaboration, and to build confidence to overcome individual challenges. Simulation scenarios are therefore frequently designed to include PAL for learners to work together in small groups so that these outcomes may be achieved, because simulation provides a practical venue for interprofessional learning and to deliver programmes at scale.

While common, it is important that PAL interactions are nonetheless deliberately designed in consideration of relevant learning outcomes such as communication, teamwork, problem solving, critical thinking and interprofessional skills. For example, learning teams may be provided with uncertain scenarios and scaffolded opportunities to explore and develop approaches to solving dilemmas together. Alternatively, learners may be grouped in diverse teams with activities focused on developing understanding, empathy and cultural humility gained from diverse perspectives and experiences of relevance to teamwork and patient/client-centred care rather than technical skill or complex problem solving. Peers can also exchange valuable feedback with one another, offering different perspectives and insights than educators or simulated participants, in turn promoting the development of feedback literacy and evaluative judgement. In doing so, learners not directly involved in the action at any given time remain actively engaged and continue learning.

PAL experiences in simulation need to be designed with psychological safety and quality learning in mind, ensuring participants' comfort to learn together rather than pressure from observation and critique. The briefing phase (see the following section on implementing placement) is essential in establishing the learning environment, and educators should also consult Chapter 4 to understand best practices.

Role of supervision

A supervisor in simulation is often referred to as a facilitator, reflecting their role in enabling a learner-centred approach. While simulation may allow for a learner-centred approach by reducing the risks to other people and organisations, it is not itself without direct physical and psychological risk to all participants and indirect risks arising from deficiencies in learning. The engagement of well-trained and supported facilitators is crucial to enhancing the safety of learners and all other participants in simulation (simulated patients/clients, staff, etc.).

To enable safe learning, facilitators typically have a central role in the briefing and debriefing/feedback phases of simulation (see the following section on implementing placement), as well as the simulation activity itself. Deliberate simulation learning strategies for these phases are set out in what follows. Facilitators may also be involved in learner preparation and evaluation/assessment.

Consistent with the role of facilitator in a learner-centred approach, it is characteristic of simulation that facilitators maintain a supportive stance whilst scaffolding their contributions to enable learners' active engagement and progressive development. In doing so, they can enable learners to 'have a go' and gain the most of simulation providing learning opportunities whereby stumbles and errors are less consequential than with real clients/patients.

Mode of delivery

Depending on the learning outcomes and chosen simulation modalities (see later in this chapter), simulation may be suited to face-to-face or online delivery. Hybrid modes – such as when students at home or a remote site use web conferencing to instruct an in-person facilitator or peer who in turn interacts with a mannequin or simulated participant – also widen opportunities for participation. For some knowledge application, communication and teamwork learning outcomes, online approaches may be as effective as face-to-face approaches whilst also reducing isolation and overcoming barriers to in-person gathering such as distance, travel time, a lack of physical space and the inaccessibility of appropriate learning spaces.

Settings for simulated placements may also vary. They are commonly implemented in higher education or clinical teaching institutions, or in dedicated simulation or clinical skills centres or repurposed learning spaces. They may also be designed 'in situ', taking place in the health workplace such as hospital ward or community centre. Increasingly, online simulated placements replicate telehealth and similar consultations, while the variety of virtual and artificial intelligence simulation platforms are supporting a new level of self-paced simulation.

Finally, simulation *modalities* vary and may include educator or peer role play, simulated patients (actors, community members or volunteer patients), masks and/or moulage to represent physical features, part-task trainers or mannequins, and VR/AR and AI systems. The chosen modality will influence uncertainty and realism achieved and therefore should consider the level of learner, learning outcomes, resources, and space and equipment (see Figure 7.1). *Role plays*, *simulated patients*, and the application of *masks and moulage* provide varying levels of uncertainty and realism applicable to developing communication skills and understanding the impacts of health conditions and their management on the whole person and significant others. Exercise physiology or physiotherapy students might role play with each other and their peers to develop skills for effective instruction and feedback on movement performance and equipment use. Occupational therapy and social work students might practice discussion of sensitive topics like suicidal ideation or violence in relationships with simulated patients, with opportunities for targeted feedback and practice while minimising risks to real healthcare users. Alternatively, a highly realistic simulated placement may involve speech pathology students attending full-time placement in an inpatient ward at the simulation centre of their university, working through their assigned lists of simulated patients portrayed by professional medical actors. *Part-task trainers* and *mannequins* provide increasingly realistic representations that are well-suited to learning intervention techniques and the management of clinical deterioration. Podiatry or dental students may undertake training in specific procedures utilising rudimentary part-task trainers prior to more traditional placements in clinic settings with real healthcare users. Physiotherapy students might practice with skills such as suctioning techniques for children in a paediatric intensive care unit (PICU) using paediatric mannequins. *VR* modalities with *AI*-guided responses may be a sound investment for training in interpersonal scenarios that may pose physical risks if performed poorly, such as the de-escalation of agitation and conflict, as learners become more proficient in more complex situations.

Planning and preparation

Significant planning and preparation are essential for implementing a successful simulated placement. In addition to typical placement preparation tasks such as creating student and staffing timetables, developing learning outcomes, scheduling opportunities and enabling assessments, there are additional considerations specific to simulation. Simulated placements rely on the cultivation of learning opportunities by creating the content, learning environment and activities. An online learning management system may be necessary to provide supporting resources and maintain patient notes/electronic medical records (EMRs). Once the modality (e.g., role play, simulated patients, mannequins, task trainers, virtual reality) and delivery mode (e.g., face to face, online, hybrid, virtual) are chosen, the experience is brought to life with scenarios and supporting materials to convey the patient situation, background, present context, simulation setting and anticipated outcomes. Delivery requires lesson plans, briefing and debriefing models and activities, simulated participant notes, facilitator notes and student materials. Technical support and equipment lists, including detailed setup requirements for mannequins or simulated participants, are crucial for smooth running and supported by practice and photos alongside written instruction.

Staff training is essential to ensure a clear understanding of simulation facilitation styles and techniques (e.g., pre-briefing, timeouts, debriefing), as well as the operational procedures of the placement. Likewise, students require upskilling to effectively learn *how* to learn in a simulated environment such as engaging with peer learning, developing reflection and feedback skills, and immersing in the scenario by suspending disbelief (known as a fiction contract; Sharma et al., 2023).

Implementing placement

Simulated placements can be designed to mimic traditional placements or concentrate on specific knowledge, skills and attitudes. But whatever the scope, typically they involve learners moving through the phases of simulation, perhaps multiple times for multiple scenarios.

Preparation for the student needs to include orientation to the learning outcomes and relevant required knowledge. *Briefing* provides learners specific orientation to the simulated placement environment and expectations, playing an essential role in establishing the psychological safety necessary for learning. Participants discuss relevant elements of the 'fiction contract' such as the limitations of the simulation and their resolution (for example, briefing how a mannequin may be unable to appear blue/cyanotic or a simulated patient unable to replicate sounds of sputum retention on auscultation and where relevant vital statistics and assessment findings are available to learners from other sources). The learners are guided through an exploration of the information sources, including medical records or correspondence, as well as the safe and effective operation of any equipment (e.g., patient handling or monitoring equipment, as well as operation of simulation-related technologies). Completed preparation work is reviewed and expected outcomes are established, along with the roles of learners and educators. Where PAL is implemented, the briefing addresses good practice points around ground rules and supportive interactions, as well as negotiating roles between team members.

During the *simulation activity*, learners typically lead the scenario and interaction. Learning strategies such as timeouts, rewinds, and team-member substitutions in the scenario may be called by either learners or facilitators to support the learning outcomes. Parts of, or complete, patient therapeutic encounters are completed, with do-overs or variations as relevant to the desired learning outcomes. Facilitators implement their training on effective prompting, redirecting and team management, as well as timely response to events affecting learning, to optimise outcomes and minimise harms.

Learner diversity, equity and inclusion

Learner-centred simulated placement design has the flexibility to incorporate intentional strategies to recognise and address the unique needs of diverse learners. For example, culturally and linguistically diverse (CALD) students may find simulation challenging and exhausting as they navigate not only the content and skill development but also the extra cognitive load of interpreting language and understanding cultural and societal norms (Attrill et al., 2020). Students with heightened levels of arousal or anxiety, or with highly discrepant academic versus interpersonal skill profiles, may benefit from scaffolded opportunities and repetition in low-stakes environments to enable success with graded activities. Students with physical and sensory disabilities, or those with different life experiences than their majority peers, may benefit from exposure to realistic settings, explicit expectations and opportunities to practice skills and strategies that they can transfer to workplace settings. Many student groups benefit from PAL in simulated placements, increasing their engagement and confidence, enabling learning through role modelling, reducing anxiety and developing interpersonal skills.

Simulated placements also afford unique opportunities to foster inclusion through the design of scenarios reflective of the diversity of the community. Factors such as age, gender, sexuality, ethnicity, socioeconomic status, health condition and cultural background can be considered to ensure inclusive learning resources. Mannequins and part-task trainers representing different ages, sexes and skin tones are increasingly available. With explicit design and trained facilitators, simulated placements may also be ideal for exploring the impacts of cultural beliefs, values and practices on patient care and communication while limiting the consequences for patients, services and students alike. Training for facilitators of simulation should therefore always include discussion around unconscious bias, cultural humility and inclusive teaching strategies.

Considerations for learner feedback and assessment

Debriefing is a critical phase of simulation to enable learning, promote consolidation and transfer of knowledge and skills, and ensure the maintenance of psychological safety. Facilitation of simulation debriefing is a unique and high-impact skill demanding facilitator training and support.

Extended *feedback* opportunities, including during debriefing sessions and with feedback from peers and simulated patients/clients (if they are part of the simulation design), are advantageous and novel features of simulation. Feedback may be provided to participants 'in action', given that scenarios can be paused, as well as 'on-action' during feedback sessions, written reports or assessments, and group debriefings. Peers offer unique perspectives and benefit themselves from observing and formulating feedback for others (see Chapter 4 for more detail on the specific benefits and good practice points for peer feedback). The patient/client perspective often provides particularly unique insights on areas such as communication and body language, use of jargon, sense of empathy and manual handling which differs from educator or peer feedback and is easier to consistently elicit than in traditional placement.

Reflection by students, which should incorporate the rich and diverse feedback available, encourages students to consolidate learning, critically analyse their experiences and identify strengths and strategies for growth. Reflections can feed forward into subsequent scenarios and self-assessment, as well as look back on a completed experience and assessment. Support to enact change and transfer learning can be scaffolded with action plans guiding goal setting and identifying additional resources or learning opportunities. Actioning feedback and reflection based on authentic experiences and feedback can be particularly motivating, encouraging the transfer of learning and preventing learning decay, whereby a 'real' experience or more traditional placement occurs soon after the simulation.

Assessment of students varies to align with learning outcomes such as clinical skills, professionalism, communication and teamwork. Opportunities for formative or summative assessments of performance include direct observation, structured assessments, self assessments and peer assessments, and/or debriefings. Given that many features of the simulation are known by design, it is frequently feasible to use rubrics to support consistent and multi-source evaluation. However, it is important to consider the tensions between the assessment of student competence and the maintenance of the psychological safety required to engage in authentic learning and feedback without fear of judgement or reprisal. In some situations, a simulated placement may justify a high-stakes summative assessment, after formative or low-stakes assessments or as a component of programmatic assessment. In other cases, it may be appropriate that the assessment of simulation remains formative in support of other learning and placement experiences or subsequent progression to programmatic assessment opportunities.

Post-placement tasks and evaluation

Evaluation and post-placement processes addressing all stakeholders – such as students, simulated patients, educators and subsequent instructors – make for a comprehensive closing of the loop. Evaluations may address effectiveness, efficiency, relevance and impact on learners, and should reflect predetermined learning outcomes and criteria around which the simulation was designed (e.g., levels of learner, resources, considerations for specific learner groups). Learning outcomes may include areas such as student performance, engagement, satisfaction, knowledge retention, skill development and behaviour change.

Specific to simulation, evaluation of relevancy, realism, effect on competency and transfer to clinical practice are helpful areas to explore. Evaluation findings should always inform continuous improvement efforts, making necessary adjustments to the programme based on feedback, and periodically re-evaluating learning outcomes and design criteria to ensure ongoing success. Well-designed simulated placements also provide a rich opportunity for a range of educational research.

With the potential that simulation can raise issues for students, simulated patients and facilitators alike, all simulation participants should be offered both adequate debriefing and options for ongoing support or further debriefing post-placement. For students, the realism of simulation and/or the implications for their learning may raise concerns or be confronting or triggering, particularly when scenarios have not gone well or to plan. For simulated patients, simulation is frequently an intense and exhausting experience. The demand for both physical and emotional authenticity, the repetition of experiences with the same or different outcomes, and the blurring of boundaries between personal and simulated experiences may result in fatigue and distress. This is particularly but not only pertinent when simulated participants portray scenarios that resonate with their own personal experiences, illness or trauma, evoking intense emotions and memories. It can also apply to those who 'voice' interactions through technologies including mannequins as much as to those who directly engage with students. For facilitators, the simulation role is dynamic and taxing, and it involves both observing and supporting others through often intense experiences. The facilitator needs to remain neutral and manage situations throughout the experience, which can lead to absorbing others' concerns and a level of vicarious stress. They, like students and simulated patients, are also potentially exposed to scenarios that have personal relevance and realism that may evoke memories and emotional reactions. This is particularly but not only pertinent to lived experience or cultural facilitators. All participant groups benefit from the opportunity for adequate debriefing that is skilfully facilitated to safely address stressors and concerns. Facilitators and other educators have this responsibility to students and simulated participants, and to each other. It is good practice to additionally offer post-placement and confidential support options, particularly as participants may not be comfortable discussing concerns in a group environment with peers or with a facilitator who may be also responsible for assessment, performance evaluation and/or employment.

Resources, funding and hidden costs

A frequently cited barrier to simulated placement uptake is cost and resourcing. Economic evaluations of simulation are complex, but research suggests real costs are not too dissimilar to more traditional placement models

(Gospodarevskaya et al., 2019). However, simulation makes evident resource demands of placements that are often distributed among stakeholders including clinicians, service providers, universities and students. Less easily counted are the benefits of simulation in terms of learning outcomes, efficiencies in delivery and the tangible and intangible costs averted through students making fewer errors with real patients (Maloney and Haines, 2016).

To design simulation for efficiency and cost-effectiveness, the building blocks of simulated placements (see Figure 7.1) can be used to guide selections. Specifically, the most realistic and feature-rich equipment and facilities are not always optimal for learning. Less expensive options may be selected or blended within a simulated placement using repurposed spaces. Peers can serve as co-facilitators or 'peer patients', benefiting in their own learning while providing the benefits of PAL and cost-effective options relative to actors as simulated patients for some situations. Likewise, patient or community volunteers may derive personal benefit while providing an educational service in a cost-effective arrangement. Other options include resource partnerships between service providers and educational institutions, sharing facilities, equipment, and facilitator and educator roles to the benefit of both students and clinicians.

The costs of simulation should not, however, be underestimated to ensure that programmes are sustainable. The initial investments in facilities and equipment need to be supported with ongoing maintenance of equipment such as mannequins, task trainers, and simulation software. Dedicated simulation technicians or support staff may be necessary to set up and operate simulation equipment, troubleshoot technical issues, and assist during simulation sessions. Optimising or integrating simulation technology with other educational technologies may also require additional investments in licences, infrastructure and ongoing support. Staff and actors incur salary expenses for their involvement but also require training to perform their roles effectively. Running expenses such as consumables (e.g., medical supplies, therapy materials or moulage materials), utilities, cleaning services, security and facility management may also be directly attributable to simulation, while other placement models may absorb these with service provision.

Capital funding for facilities, equipment and training may be available from various bodies invested in the impacts that simulation may make to learning outcomes and the future competence of health professionals and thereby public safety. Innovations are making lower-cost models of simulated placements more accessible. Additional efficiencies may also be gained by sharing expenses in facilities, equipment and learning material development across programmes or between simulation and other learning or service provision objectives.

PRACTICE EXAMPLE 1

At the University of Sydney in Australia, occupational therapy, physiotherapy and speech pathology students each engage in well-established, immersive, face-to-face simulated placements prior to their first traditional placements. The specific simulated placement models are course-specific, with each student completing five days scheduled either consecutively or across a teaching session. The universal aim of these novice-level placement designs is to support the translation of classroom knowledge and skills to the development of foundational clinical competencies required for safe and effective practice. The programmes are held in dedicated simulation facilities at the university, including mock hospital wards, rehabilitation gyms, private treatment rooms and breakout tutorial areas. The programme is high fidelity whereby the environment represents authentic clinical practice areas, and professional medical actors are employed as simulated patients portraying patient scenarios adapted from authentic situations. The programme progression mimics the demands and experiences of a typical placement experience including patient file review, liaising with nursing staff, assessing, and treating patients, documentation of sessions, in-services, and consideration of the multidisciplinary team involvement in patient management. Students receive formal and informal feedback from peers, facilitators and simulated patients, and they engage in self-reflection. Students must pass a longitudinal assessment of their performance in the programme to progress to the following placement.

Students work in small groups (typically 4–5 students) with the direct supervision of a practice educator – who is sought from clinical practice – assigned to each group. The educators adopt a predominantly hands-off facilitation style, allowing students to take the lead in sessions. Typical simulation-style facilitation strategies are adopted, allowing educators or students to call a timeout or rewind in the scenarios. Actors are trained in the social background story of the scenario, as well as the physical presentation. Facilitators are briefed in how to support students in this placement model, and students are briefed on how to best learn in simulation. Students and facilitators cycle through a daily programme of patient file review and preparation, nurse consultation, patient encounter, debrief and documentation, with ample repetition akin to traditional placements.

Underperforming students not at the foundational level of competency at the end of the week have their course progression paused. These students enter a remediation programme that may involve meeting with simulation programme leads and creating learning plans, engaging with the university's learning centre, participating in immersive simulation remediation, undertaking self-study or volunteer work, and meeting with the cohort student liaison academic before returning to repeat the formal simulated placement.

Clinical educators at external placement sites report that students are better prepared after completing the simulation placement, more confident and ready for real clinical practice.

PRACTICE EXAMPLE 2

A cross-institutional interprofessional learning (IPL) online simulation programme is being piloted among several universities with health professional training programmes in Australia. Interdisciplinary teams are comprised of intermediate (typically second-year) students from dietetics, medicine, occupational therapy, physiotherapy, social work and speech pathology, coming together to enhance professional and interprofessional identity through greater understanding of each other's roles. Each team is assigned a simulation scenario on which they collaborate to strengthen their team patient clinical management skills. Students connect online via a common learning management site (LMS). They have access to videorecorded vignettes of the patient as portrayed by professional actors and accompanying electronic medical records.

The teams spend time online (usually 3–4 hours) in their groups establishing the patient priorities and key impairments and formulating a tailored team-based management plan. Educators are available online for consultation as needed, but student teams work independently. Each team then submits a written or videorecorded summary of their patient management plan with an emphasis on patient impairments and priorities rather than discipline specific tasks. Educators provide feedback on each submission via the LMS.

The cross-institutional nature of the model authentically reflects the nature of healthcare workplaces and instils students early with skills and attitudes that enable interprofessional working. The online collaboration provides accessibility for students who might otherwise have extremely limited IPL opportunities, such as those on campuses with few other health disciplines or those who may be in rural and remote areas or overseas. Unsurprisingly, a challenge to this model is scheduling and managing student attendance changes to support a good mix of disciplines in each student group. Scenarios also need to be developed suitable for a wide variety of professions to engage authentically with, and at a complexity level that suits learners. Clinician reference groups in the development phase of this programme assisted ensuring scenario appropriateness. This simulation experience currently runs as a formative learning opportunity only. Rubrics guide quality feedback on submissions as feedback for learning only.

CONCLUSION

This chapter has explored simulated placement models. Simulated placements are built on pedagogical theories and possess a growing evidence base supporting their implementation and positive effect on student learning. These models provide flexibility in their design that can be tailored to different learner groups and constraints. Simulated placements offer flexible and controllable learning experiences for students that may present a safer opportunity to develop clinical skills that can be tailored to specific educational needs. Therefore, simulated placements offer features that centre the student at the core of the learning experience. Practice examples highlighted different modalities through which simulated placements can be delivered and to meet a variety of learning objectives. Simulated placements require considerable planning and resourcing; however, many low-cost options are demonstrating considerable benefit for student learning.

REFERENCES

Alanazi, A. A. and Nicholson, N. (2023). The use of simulation in audiology education: A systematic review. *American Journal of Audiology*, *32*(3), pp. 640–656. https://doi.org/10.1044/2023_AJA-23-00054

Alanzi, A. A., Nicholson, N. and Thomas, S. (2017). The use of simulation training to improve knowledge, skills, and confidence among healthcare students: A systematic review. *Internet Journal of Allied Health Sciences and Practice*, *15*(3), Article 2.

Attrill, S., Lincoln, M. and McAllister, S. (2020, March). International students in professional placements: Supervision strategies for positive learning experiences. *International Journal of Language & Communication Disorders*, *55*(2), pp. 243–254.

Beshir, S. A., Mohamed, A. P., Soorya, A., Goh, S. S. L., El-Labadd, E. M., Hussain, N. and Said, A. S. (2022). Virtual patient simulation in pharmacy education: A systematic review. *Pharmacy Education*, *22*(1), pp. 954–970.

Bloom, B. S. (1968). Learning for mastery. Instruction and curriculum. Regional Education Laboratory for the Carolinas and Virginia, Topical Papers and Reprints, Number 1. *Evaluation Comment*, *1*(2), p. n2.

Bogossian, F. E., et al. (2019). Locating "gold standard" evidence for simulation as a substitute for clinical practice in prelicensure health professional education: A systematic review. *Journal of Clinical Nursing*, *28*(21–22), pp. 3759–3775. https://doi.org/10.1111/jocn.14965

Cant, R. P. and Cooper, S. J. (2010). Simulation-based learning in nurse education: Systematic review. *Journal of Advanced Nursing*, *66*(1), pp. 3–15.

Chen, F. Q., Leng, Y. F., Ge, J. F., Wang, D. W., Li, C., Chen, B. and Sun, Z. L. (2020). Effectiveness of virtual reality in nursing education: Meta-analysis. *Journal of Medical Internet Research*, *22*(9), p. e18290.

Chua, J. Y. X., Ang, E., Lau, S. T. L. and Shorey, S. (2021). Effectiveness of simulation-based interventions at improving empathy among healthcare students: A systematic review and meta-analysis. *Nurse Education Today*, *104*, p. 105000.

Cook, D. A., et al. (2011). Technology-enhanced simulation for health professions education: A systematic review and meta-analysis. *Journal of the American Medical Association*, *306*(9). https://doi.org/10.1001/jama.2011.1234

Cook, D. A., et al. (2012). Comparative effectiveness of technology-enhanced simulation versus other instructional methods: A systematic review and meta-analysis. *Simulation in Healthcare: The Journal of the Society for Simulation in Healthcare*, *7*(5), pp. 308–320. https://doi.org/10.1097/SIH.0b013e3182614f95

Dalwood, N., et al. (2020). Students as patients: A systematic review of peer simulation in health care professional education. *Medical Education*, *54*(5), pp. 387–399. https://doi.org/10.1111/medu.14058

Diaz-Navarro, C., et al. (2024). The ASPiH standards – 2023: Guiding simulation-based practice in health and care. *International Journal of Healthcare Simulation*, pp. 1–12. https://doi.org/10.54531/nyvm5886

Foronda, C. L., Fernandez-Burgos, M., Nadeau, C., Kelley, C. N. and Henry, M. N. (2020). Virtual simulation in nursing education: A systematic review spanning 1996 to 2018. *Simulation in Healthcare*, *15*(1), pp. 46–54.

Gaba, D. M. (2004). The future vision of simulation in health care. *Quality and Safety in Health Care*, *13*(Supplement 1), pp. i2–i10. https://doi.org/10.1136/qshc.2004.009878

Gormley, G. J. and Murphy, P. (2023). When I say . . . simulation. *Medical Education*, p. medu.15165. https://doi.org/10.1111/medu.15165

Gospodarevskaya, E., Carter, R., Imms, C., Chu, E. M. Y., Nicola-Richmond, K., Gribble, N., . . . and Chen, G. (2019). Economic evaluation of simulated and traditional clinical placements in occupational therapy education. *Australian Occupational Therapy Journal*, *66*(3), pp. 369–379.

Hegland, P. A., Aarlie, H., Strømme, H. and Jamtvedt, G. (2017). Simulation-based training for nurses: Systematic review and meta-analysis. *Nurse Education Today*, *54*, pp. 6–20.

Hill, A. E., Ward, E., Heard, R., McAllister, S., McCabe, P., Penman, A., . . . and Walters, J. (2021). Simulation can replace part of speech-language pathology placement time: A randomised controlled trial. *International Journal of Speech-Language Pathology*, *23*(1), pp. 92–102.

Imms, C., Froude, E., Chu, E. M. Y., Sheppard, L., Darzins, S., Guinea, S., . . . and Mathieu, E. (2018). Simulated versus traditional occupational therapy placements: A randomised controlled trial. *Australian Occupational Therapy Journal*, *65*(6), pp. 556–564.

Javaherian, M., Dabbaghipour, N., Mafinejad, M. K., Ghotbi, N., Khakneshin, A. A. and Moghadam, B. A. (2020). The role of simulated patient in physiotherapy education: A review article. *Journal of Modern Rehabilitation*, *14*(2), pp. 69–80.

Ketterer, S.-J., et al. (2020). Simulated versus traditional therapeutic radiography placements: A randomised controlled trial. *Radiography*, *26*(2), pp. 140–146. https://doi.org/10.1016/j.radi.2019.10.005

Kneebone, R., Nestel, D., Wetzel, C., Black, S., Jacklin, R., Aggarwal, R., . . . and Darzi, A. (2006). The human face of simulation: Patient-focused simulation training. *Academic Medicine*, *81*(10), pp. 919–924.

Kononowicz, A. A., Woodham, L. A., Edelbring, S., Stathakarou, N., Davies, D., Saxena, N., . . . and Zary, N. (2019). Virtual patient simulations in health professions education: Systematic review and meta-analysis by the digital health education collaboration. *Journal of Medical Internet Research*, *21*(7), p. e14676.

Kourgiantakis, T., Sewell, K. M., Hu, R., Logan, J. and Bogo, M. (2020). Simulation in social work education: A scoping review. *Research on Social Work Practice*, *30*(4), pp. 433–450.

Larue, C., Pepin, J. and Allard, É. (2015). Simulation in preparation or substitution for clinical placement: A systematic review of the literature. *Journal of Nursing Education and Practice*, *5*(9), p. 132. https://doi.org/10.5430/jnep.v5n9p132

MacBean, N., Theodoros, D., Davidson, B. and Hill, A. E. (2013). Simulated learning environments in speech-language pathology: An Australian response. *International Journal of Speech-Language Pathology*, *15*(3), pp. 345–357.

Maloney, S. and Haines, T. (2016). Issues of cost-benefit and cost-effectiveness for simulation in health professions education. *Advances in Simulation*, *1*, pp. 1–6.

Marion-Martins, A. D. and Pinho, D. L. (2020). Interprofessional simulation effects for healthcare students: A systematic review and meta-analysis. *Nurse Education Today*, *94*, p. 104568.

Mori, B., Carnahan, H. and Herold, J. (2015). Use of simulation learning experiences in physical therapy entry-to-practice curricula: A systematic review. *Physiotherapy Canada*, *67*(2), pp. 194–202.

Motola, I., Devine, L. A., Chung, H. S., Sullivan, J. E. and Issenberg, S. B. (2013). Simulation in healthcare education: A best evidence practical guide. AMEE Guide No. 82. *Medical Teacher*, *35*(10), pp. e1511–e1530.

Pritchard, S. A., Blackstock, F. C., Nestel, D. and Keating, J. L. (2016). Simulated patients in physical therapy education: Systematic review and meta-analysis. *Physical Therapy*, *96*(9), pp. 1342–1353.

Rezayi, S., Shahmoradi, L., Ghotbi, N., Choobsaz, H., Yousefi, M. H., Pourazadi, S. and Ardali, Z. R. (2022). Computerized simulation education on physiotherapy students' skills and knowledge: A systematic review. *BioMed Research International*.

Royal College of Occupational Therapists. (2019). *Learning and Development Standards for Pre-Registration Education*. London: Royal College of Occupational Therapists.

Sezgin, M. G. and Bektas, H. (2023). Effectiveness of interprofessional simulation-based education programs to improve teamwork and communication for students in the healthcare profession: A systematic review and meta-analysis of randomized controlled trials. *Nurse Education Today*, *120*, p. 105619. https://doi.org/10.1016/j.nedt.2022.105619

Sharma, H., Patil, A. D. and Baviskar, A. (2023). Fiction contract: Its importance in simulation-based medical education. *International Journal of Basic & Clinical Pharmacology*, *12*(5), p. 766.

Squires, K., et al. (2022). Mapping simulated-based learning experiences incorporated into professional placements in allied health programs: A scoping review. *Simulation in Healthcare: The Journal of the Society for Simulation in Healthcare*, *17*(6), pp. 403–415. https://doi.org/10.1097/SIH.0000000000000627

Watson, K., Wright, A., Morris, N., McMeeken, J., Rivett, D., Blackstock, F., . . . and Jull, G. (2012). Can simulation replace part of clinical time? Two parallel randomised controlled trials. *Medical Education*, *46*(7), pp. 657–667.

Watts, P. I., Rossler, K., Bowler, F., Miller, C., Charnetski, M., Decker, S., . . . and Hallmark, B. (2021). Onward and upward: Introducing the healthcare simulation standards of best practice. *Clinical Simulation in Nursing*, *58*, pp. 1–4.

Chapter 8

Role-emerging placements

Emma Green, Anita Volkert and Rowenna Harrison

CHAPTER OVERVIEW

This chapter explores role-emerging placements in allied health education, providing a comprehensive overview of their definition, rationale and evidence base. Unlike traditional placements, role-emerging placements place students in non-traditional settings without an established allied health professional, fostering autonomy, innovation and interdisciplinary collaboration. The chapter examines the benefits of role-emerging placements, including enhanced professional identity, problem-solving skills and increased employability, as well as challenges such as the absence of direct supervision and variability in placement experiences. Drawing on key literature and real-world case examples, this chapter outlines best practices for designing, implementing and evaluating role-emerging placements to maximise student learning and professional development. Ultimately, role-emerging placements serve as a transformative approach to allied health education, equipping students with the skills needed to navigate and contribute to evolving healthcare landscapes.

CHAPTER OBJECTIVES

The objectives of this chapter are the following.

- A definition and rationale for role-emerging placements to support allied health practice-based learning.
- An overview of the evidence base for role-emerging placements outlining the benefits and challenges of developing and implementing role-emerging placements.
- Considerations of the design principles of setting up, implementing and evaluating a role-emerging placement.
- Real-world case examples of role-emerging placements.

DOI: 10.4324/9781003411765-8

INTRODUCTION

Role-emerging placements in allied health provide students with practice-based learning opportunities in non-traditional settings where there is no existing allied health professional in that role. Designed to foster autonomy, innovation and decision-making, these placements integrate allied health services into new or underdeveloped areas of practice, addressing the needs of individuals, groups and communities (Overton et al., 2009). Unlike traditional placements – where students work under direct supervision in hospitals or clinics – role-emerging placements take place in diverse settings where allied health professionals may not yet be established (Clarke et al., 2014), such as community centres, homeless shelters, schools, prisons, workplaces or non-governmental organisations (NGOs). This model enables students to take a broader approach to health and wellbeing, addressing structural, systemic and societal factors that influence overall health outcomes.

A key feature of role-emerging placements is student-driven learning, requiring adaptability, problem solving, and advocacy skills to establish and demonstrate the value of their profession in new environments (Cooper and Raine, 2009). While students receive external supervision from a university-appointed allied health professional, such as a faculty member or a registered practitioner providing long-arm supervision, day-to-day support and mentorship typically comes from on-site supervisors within the service.

These placements can be uni-professional or interprofessional, though they are often structured as peer-learning experiences whereby students work in pairs or groups. This collaborative approach enhances teamwork, fosters peer support and encourages students to push professional boundaries while addressing service gaps to meet the unmet needs of communities. Role-emerging placements help shape adaptable, forward-thinking professionals, equipping them with the skills and experience needed to navigate the evolving landscape of health and social care (Clarke et al., 2014).

EVIDENCE BASE FOR ROLE-EMERGING PLACEMENTS

The evidence supporting role-emerging placements has been steadily growing for many years. In some professions, such as occupational therapy, these placements have been in use since the 1970s in countries like Canada, the United States and Australia, gaining momentum during the 1990s (Bossers et al., 1997). For other allied health professions, however, interest in role-emerging placements has emerged more recently, driven by the increasing demand for placement opportunities, addressing increasing numbers of students in the sector, but also for the exposure to wider contexts and enhanced skill set these placements can provide (Kyte et al., 2018). Much of the research to date has focused on the experiences of learners and practice educators within allied health professions, with a strong emphasis on qualitative studies in occupational therapy. This is due to the long-standing implementation of role-emerging placements in that field (Overton et al., 2009; Clarke et al., 2014; Lau and Ravenek, 2019).

In occupational therapy specifically, three key literature reviews have examined role-emerging placements. The first, conducted by Overton et al. (2009), took a broad approach, reviewing research and expert opinions on new and emerging placement models. This review considered perspectives from learners, educators, other health professionals and organisations, identifying both benefits and challenges. The authors concluded that role-emerging placements push the profession beyond traditional boundaries, fostering growth and expanding opportunities beyond its existing scope. A later review by Clarke et al. (2014) focused on the UK context, analysing the rationale behind and development of role-emerging placements. This critical review identified both strengths and limitations, highlighting three main benefits when placements were well-designed: (1) raising the profile of occupational therapy; (2) increasing students' political awareness; and (3) enhancing learners' self-confidence and professional identity. More recently, Lau and Ravenek (2019) conducted a scoping review that specifically examined students' perspectives on role-emerging placements. Their findings underscored both the benefits and challenges of this learning model, particularly emphasising its value across all stages of education, including for novice learners. The review concluded that role-emerging placements play a crucial role in fostering both personal and professional development.

Benefits of role-emerging placements

Most literature on role-emerging placements focuses on the experiences, benefits and challenges associated with this placement model – and as a result, these aspects are well documented. One of the key advantages of role-emerging placements is that they offer students real-world opportunities to engage in person-centred practice (Lau and Ravenek, 2019). By working directly with individuals, groups or communities – regardless of disability – students step outside the dominant medical model, building meaningful relationships and addressing needs in a holistic manner (Overton et al., 2009; Dancza et al., 2013; Clarke et al., 2014; Lau and Ravenek, 2019). A defining feature of these placements is their peer-learning structure, whereby students work in pairs or groups, either within their own profession or in an interprofessional capacity. Research suggests that this collaborative approach enhances teamwork and communication skills, supporting both learning and practice development (Lau and Ravenek, 2019).

From a professional development perspective, role-emerging placements provide a unique learning environment. Entering a setting without an established allied health professional challenges students to develop strong professional identities, helping them refine their senses of purpose, direction and clarity in their chosen field (Warren, 2014; Clarke et al., 2015a). The literature indicates that in the absence of an on-site supervisor, students engage more deeply and critically with reflective practice, using this as a tool to navigate their learning and professional growth (Cooper and Raine, 2009; Dancza et al., 2013). This independent learning experience is also linked to increased self-confidence in future practice. Without the constant validation of a supervisor, students develop problem-solving abilities, professional reasoning and decision-making skills, which are essential for clinical and community-based work (Overton et al., 2009; Clarke et al., 2014; Lau and Ravenek, 2019).

Additionally, there is evidence that students who complete role-emerging placements feel better prepared for job interviews, often perceiving their experience as an advantage in securing employment (Clarke et al., 2015a). These placements also expose students to a broader range of career possibilities, particularly in emerging areas of practice, expanding their post-graduate opportunities and long-term career success (Thew et al., 2018; Syed and Duncan, 2019).

Challenges and limitations identified in the literature

The literature highlights several challenges associated with role-emerging placements. One of the most cited concerns is the absence of on-site professional supervision, which has been shown to heighten student anxieties and uncertainties (Dancza et al., 2013; Clarke et al., 2014; Clarke et al., 2015b). However, as this is a well-recognised limitation, best practices emphasise the importance of designing placements with clear supervision structures, ensuring that students receive the necessary guidance and support (Clarke et al., 2015b). To address this challenge, role-emerging placements are often structured around peer learning, enabling students to support each other while complementing the guidance of an on-site mentor – who is typically not an allied health professional – and an external, professionally qualified supervisor (Thew et al., 2008; Cooper and Raine, 2009; Thew et al., 2011; Thomas and Rodger, 2011). Additionally, setting clear expectations from the outset is crucial in reducing student anxieties. Properly framing the placement experience helps prepare learners by shifting their perspective from a traditional medical model to a holistic, preventive and health-promoting social model of disability (Dancza et al., 2013). To achieve this, situated experiential learning supported by reflection is key to facilitating and optimising student learning (Dancza et al., 2013). Indeed, it could be argued this challenge can operate as a strength, as students learn to self-manage on these placements (Mattila et al., 2018).

Another challenge noted in the literature is the variability among placement sites (Clarke et al., 2014). Differences in service-user contact, access to resources, and the overall structure of each placement can create inconsistencies in the student experience. However, careful selection of placement sites, along with clearly defined learning outcomes and expectations for both students and service providers, can help mitigate these concerns. By ensuring well-structured placements, students can have a more fulfilling and enriching learning experience.

DESIGN PRINCIPLES OF ROLE-EMERGING PLACEMENTS

Role-emerging placements need to be well-designed to ensure that students receive clear role definitions, structured supervision and adequate support to thrive in non-traditional settings. A carefully planned approach addresses potential challenges such as role uncertainty, ethical dilemmas and student isolation, promoting successful integration into host organisations and ensuring meaningful community impact. Additionally, well-designed placements include mechanisms for ongoing evaluation and feedback, allowing for continuous improvement and alignment with both educational goals and the evolving needs of the healthcare landscape. This thoughtful structure maximises the effectiveness of the placement experience for students, supervisors and host organisations alike. See Table 8.1 for summary of design principles to support the development of role-emerging placements.

Rationale for role-emerging placements

The primary rationale for integrating role-emerging placements in allied health is the unique opportunity they provide to expand professional practice and contribute to health and wellbeing at a population level. These placements encourage allied health professionals to extend their roles beyond traditional service boundaries, fostering growth and innovation in emerging areas of practice (Clarke et al., 2014). From a service perspective, role-emerging placements add value by enabling students to

Table 8.1 Design principles of role-emerging placements

Rationale for choice of model of placement	• Role-emerging placements broaden allied health professionals' practice beyond traditional settings, support underserved communities and help universities address placement shortages. • Role-emerging placements enhance self-directed learning, creativity, leadership and problem solving, while also strengthening students' professional identity, communication and teamwork skills. • Role-emerging placements emphasise health promotion and community engagement, and they prepare students to meet modern healthcare needs with adaptability and a strengths-based approach.
Can the placement be supported as PAL?	• Role-emerging placements typically are delivered as PAL placements to optimise learning and support for students. • Role-emerging peer-assisted learning fosters mutual support, critical thinking and professional growth by encouraging students to learn from each other while navigating less structured, real-world healthcare environments.
Approach to supervision	• Effective supervision in role-emerging placements relies on clearly defined roles and collaboration between external supervisors and on-site mentors to ensure students receive consistent guidance and achieve learning outcomes. • University-appointed allied health professionals provide remote supervision through regular check-ins, reflective tasks, case discussions and targeted feedback to guide students' learning and professional development. • Non-allied health staff (e.g., teachers, community leaders) offer daily support and workplace integration, and facilitate interprofessional learning, ensuring students are embedded in the organisational environment.
Mode of delivery	• Role-emerging placements can be in person, hybrid or fully online, enabling access to diverse settings, including rural and international locations.
Planning and preparation	• Success depends on strong university–host partnerships, defined student roles, formal agreements and well-planned supervision and mentoring structures. • Universities must provide training on professional roles, ethics, cultural competence and reflective practice to equip students for self-directed learning. • Clear learning objectives, competency frameworks and structured feedback tools (e.g., journals, evaluations) ensure student growth and placement quality.

Table 8.1 continued

Implementing placement	• Successful integration into non-traditional healthcare settings involves orientation programmes, role workshops and interprofessional collaboration, empowering students to define and lead projects. • Regular feedback, reflective practice and professional development workshops, along with networking opportunities, support student learning and career exploration. • Continuous assessment through self-reflection, supervisor feedback and host organisation evaluations ensures placement success and addresses challenges like role uncertainty, ethical issues and student isolation.
Post-placement	• Feedback from students, supervisors and host organisations helps assess the effectiveness of role-emerging placements, identify challenges and make adjustments to enhance future placements and ensure alignment with educational and community needs.

deliver preventive health and wellbeing interventions to underserved communities and populations. Universities also benefit from these placements, as they provide alternative solutions to meet regulatory placement requirements, particularly in the face of well-documented placement capacity challenges (Deaves et al., 2024). For students, the benefits are numerous, helping them develop essential professional skills and experiences that enhance their readiness for future practice.

When designed effectively, role-emerging placements can address key learning outcomes, including the following.

• **Encouraging self-directed learning, creativity, problem solving and leadership**: Without an on-site supervisor, students must critically assess client needs, apply problem-solving skills and seek guidance from external supervisors and interdisciplinary teams (Clarke et al., 2014). The absence of established practices requires learners to think creatively and adapt to their environment, fostering entrepreneurial skills and innovative thinking. This process enhances decision-making abilities, resilience and confidence in professional practice.
• **Developing a stronger professional identity**: Role-emerging placements challenge students to educate other professionals about their discipline, strengthening professional advocacy and role definition (Clarke et al., 2015a; Warren, 2014). This experience helps learners develop a clear sense of professional identity and purpose.

- **Enhancing communication and teamwork skills**: By collaborating with non-allied health professionals, students refine their communication and team-work abilities. This interprofessional exposure prepares them for multidiscipli-nary collaboration in real-world practice, an essential skill in modern healthcare settings.

Another key driver of role-emerging placements is their strong community focus, emphasising preventive care and health promotion. These experiences encourage students to adopt a proactive approach to healthcare, working within communities to build on existing strengths and resources rather than solely addressing deficits. This broader perspective equips learners to extend the scope of their professional roles, fostering adaptability and preparing them to meet the evolving demands of the healthcare landscape (Syed and Duncan, 2019).

Approach to supervision with role-emerging placement

Supervision in role-emerging placements differs significantly from traditional clinical placements due to the absence of an on-site allied health professional. Instead, students receive external supervision from university-appointed supervisors and on-site mentorship from professionals within the placement organisation, such as social workers, teachers or community leaders (Clarke et al., 2014). To ensure that students receive sufficient guidance, feedback and professional development opportunities in these autonomous and non-traditional settings, supervision must be well structured and clearly defined.

External supervision from an allied health professional

Since no allied health professional is present on-site, external supervision is the primary model used in role-emerging placements. A university-based clinical educator or an external allied health supervisor provides regular remote or long-arm supervision, ensuring that students meet their learning outcomes (Overton et al., 2009).

To optimise this support and guidance, the following key features are recommended from external supervisors.

- **Scheduled check-ins**: Supervisors conduct weekly or bi-weekly meetings (either in person or via telehealth) to provide structured supervision, feedback and support.

- **Student reflection and self-assessment**: Students engage in structured reflective practice, maintaining learning journals with clear, directed tasks. Setting explicit expectations for these reflective activities helps scaffold their learning and supports deeper professional growth.
- **Case discussions and problem solving**: Routine discussions of clinical scenarios and ethical dilemmas with external supervisors help students build confidence, refine their reasoning skills and develop professional decision-making abilities. Over time, this process strengthens their professional identity and ability to navigate complex situations independently.
- **Skill development and feedback**: Supervisors guide students through cycles of action and reflection, supporting the development of problem solving, leadership and interprofessional collaboration skills. Students are encouraged to reflect on both successes and areas for improvement, setting clear learning action plans aligned with placement expectations.

On-site mentorship (non-allied health staff)

Although students do not receive direct on-site supervision from an allied health professional, they are often mentored by professionals within the organisation who provide valuable non-clinical guidance (Clarke et al., 2014). These mentors play a crucial role in integrating students into the workplace, facilitating interprofessional learning, and supporting their day-to-day placement experience. To ensure a successful mentorship experience, universities should provide adequate training for placement mentors, so that they understand the expectations and needs of allied health students.

Key features of on-site mentorship include the following.

- **Daily point of contact**: A designated mentor provides daily check-ins to monitor student wellbeing, register attendance and offer immediate support.
- **Integration into the workplace**: Mentors help students understand organisational culture and policies, ensuring proper induction and orientation, including health and safety procedures.
- **Interprofessional learning**: Students are encouraged to collaborate with professionals outside their field, broadening their scope of practice and strengthening interdisciplinary teamwork skills.
- **Practical support and advocacy**: On-site mentors ensure students have access to necessary resources, service users and internal support networks, helping them successfully complete placement activities and achieve their learning outcomes.

The role of peer learning

Supervision in role-emerging placements is further reinforced by peer learning, a critical component widely acknowledged in literature (Lau and Ravenek, 2019). Working in pairs or small groups, students engage in the following.

• Sharing problem-solving strategies.
• Providing emotional support and resilience.
• Exchanging ideas and develop creative solutions to meet learning objectives.

This collaborative approach not only enhances the learning experience but also strengthens professional confidence, teamwork and adaptability.

Mode of delivery of role-emerging placements

Role-emerging placements, with their diverse nature, offer a flexible mode of delivery that can be in person, hybrid or fully online. This flexibility is particularly valuable in extending opportunities beyond traditional health and social care settings, especially when reaching remote or rural locations. Whether students are participating in person or virtually, the model is adaptable to various environments, ensuring accessibility across geographic barriers. The long-arm supervision approach further supports this flexibility, allowing learners to be distanced from both their supervisor and the service itself while still receiving valuable guidance online. This adaptability not only facilitates local placements but also paves the way for a truly global approach to role-emerging placements, opening opportunities for students and communities worldwide. For example, Glasgow Caledonian University (GCU) partnered with Think Pacific to provide a unique internationally focused role-emerging placement experience for occupational therapy students during the post-pandemic years of 2021–2023. This placement utilised the remote internship model developed by Think Pacific, requiring students to work with mentors from Think Pacific on a range of pre-prepared projects submitted to Think Pacific from various government and third sector agencies in Fiji. Over a six-week full-time block placement, students worked online, as individuals and within small groups and teams, using the software diary/organiser and messaging team tool Slack to communicate and plan their days and weeks with Think Pacific staff and mentors, and standard university communications to contact their faculty appointed long-arm supervisor, who provided daily check-ins as well as weekly supervision. Students utilised the following 5D Think Pacific approach to provide structure to the placement.

1. **Discover**: Learning about Fiji, the organisation, self-leadership and how the organisation supports Fiji's National Development Plan and aligns with the United Nations Sustainable Development Goals.

2. **Discussion**: Engage in discussions with NGO staff and fellow students to deepen understanding.
3. **Decide**: Choose which project to focus on.
4. **Design**: Create project; this might mean designing reports, PowerPoints, research or online campaigns.
5. **Deliver**: Present the final project to Think Pacific's senior management team and the attached partner organisation.

(Think Pacific, n.d.)

Students worked on wide-ranging public health projects such as sustainable menstrual care, reducing domestic violence rates, suicide prevention, water sanitation and funding for early-years education. The experience was transformative and opened students' eyes to working in public health, the international sector and advanced research positions. Think Pacific's strong focus on the importance of cultural immersion and competence through the 'Discover' phase – as well as the need for projects to be relevant and sustainable through their own procurement process, along with long-arm supervision from a registered allied health professional and the facilitation of positive student teamwork – ensured the success of these placements. This placement has since been adopted by other occupational therapy programmes within Scotland.

Planning and preparation for role-emerging placements

Role-emerging placements require careful planning of several considerations. The success of a role-emerging placement starts with strategic partnerships between universities and host organisations. Identifying suitable sites that align with allied health objectives is essential, with potential placements spanning community-based settings, schools, aged care facilities and non-profits (Overton et al., 2009). Establishing these partnerships requires proactive engagement with key stakeholders to clarify expectations, address concerns and create mutually beneficial learning opportunities (Overton et al., 2009). Given that role-emerging placements do not have an established allied health professional on site, it is crucial to define clear student roles to ensure alignment with service needs and learning outcomes (Clarke et al., 2014). A memorandum of understanding or service agreement formalises these agreements, outlining responsibilities, resources required, supervision structures and expected outcomes. It would also be required for relevant insurance and health and safety procedures to be considered and in place. This can include not only clarification of work-related insurances but also purchasing of professional liability insurance by the learners.

In setting up the placement, there needs to be clear and explicit discussion in relation to supervision structures. Clear expectations need to be set with potential services regarding on-site mentoring and expectations for daily support and induction, ensuring that the service has capacity for this level of support. The university also needs to make relevant and considered plans for the professional supervision, whether that is resourced via university or faculty staff or from commissioned allied health professionals. This will require consideration of resources to support this and relevant training for both professional supervisors and on-site mentors.

To thrive in a self-directed role-emerging placement, students must be well-prepared before their role-emerging placement begins. Universities should provide pre-placement training that emphasises role definition, interprofessional collaboration, ethical considerations and reflective practice (Overton et al., 2009). Placement preparation focused on scope of practice helps students establish clear professional roles in non-traditional settings and helps alleviate learner anxieties (Clarke et al., 2015b). Training in ethical and professional considerations such as confidentiality, consent and cultural competence ensures students navigate complex real-world challenges with confidence. Furthermore, given the autonomous nature of role-emerging placements, structured learning objectives and a competency framework are essential to guide student development and assessment. Additionally, structured guidance on self-directed learning and reflective practice encourages students to set learning goals, document experiences and critically assess their growth (Clarke et al., 2019). To maintain educational rigour and ensure a valuable student experience, effective assessment and feedback mechanisms must be embedded. A combination of reflective journals, supervisor evaluations, self-assessments and project-based assessments helps track progress and facilitate continuous improvement (Clarke et al., 2019).

Implementation of role-emerging placements

Integrating students into non-traditional healthcare settings is essential for the success of role-emerging placements. To ensure smooth integration, structured orientation programmes play a vital role in introducing students to the organisation's policies, culture and team members (Clarke et al., 2014). Additionally, role establishment workshops help students develop confidence in defining their professional roles, allowing them to feel empowered and well prepared (Clarke et al., 2015b). Interprofessional relationships are crucial in these placements, as they encourage collaboration with staff from various disciplines, fostering a deeper understanding of the healthcare ecosystem. Furthermore, students should be encouraged to take initiative by identifying needs, proposing solutions and leading projects, which enhances their sense of ownership and professional development (Overton et al., 2009).

Ongoing support and professional development are crucial in role-emerging placements, helping students thrive in their roles. Reflective practice and self-directed learning are key components, encouraging students to maintain learning journals and engage in guided reflection to track their progress (Clarke et al., 2019). Regular feedback and mid-placement reviews ensure that students are meeting their learning objectives and receiving necessary guidance (Rodger et al., 2009). To further enhance their professional growth, students should participate in ethical and professional development workshops, addressing critical issues such as confidentiality, cultural competence and ethical decision-making (Clarke et al., 2014). Additionally, providing networking opportunities and career development initiatives allows students to connect with professionals in emerging practice areas, exploring future career pathways (Syed and Duncan, 2019).

To ensure the continuous success of role-emerging placements, monitoring, evaluation and feedback are essential components. Students should engage in self-assessments, reflecting on their personal and professional growth throughout the placement (Lau and Ravenek, 2019). Supervisor feedback reports are crucial for assessing clinical reasoning, leadership and communication skills, offering students valuable insights for improvement (Clarke et al., 2014). Host organisations also provide feedback on student impact and placement effectiveness, which helps evaluate the success of the placement from the organisation's perspective.

Implementing role-emerging placements comes with unique challenges that require proactive problem solving. One common issue is the lack of an allied health professional on site, which can be addressed by establishing clear external supervision and structured student role definitions (Rodger et al., 2009). To combat uncertainty in role definition, pre-placement training focused on role establishment is essential (Clarke et al., 2014). Ethical and professional challenges can be mitigated by providing supervision and guidance on ethical decision-making and workplace adaptability (Clarke et al., 2019). Potential student isolation can be alleviated through peer support groups and virtual check-ins, helping students stay connected and supported (Lau et al., 2019). Additionally, limited understanding of allied health within host organisations can be addressed by offering educational materials and training sessions for staff, ensuring a more comprehensive integration of students into their roles (Overton et al., 2009).

Post-placement for role-emerging placements

Post-placement evaluation of role-emerging placements is essential for assessing the effectiveness and impact of these unique learning experiences. This evaluation involves collecting feedback from various stakeholders, including students, external supervisors and host organisations. Students engage in reflective practice through self-assessments, identifying strengths, challenges and areas for improvement (Clarke et al., 2014). Supervisors provide insights into the student's clinical reasoning, communication, leadership and teamwork skills, offering constructive feedback for future development (Rodger et al., 2009). Host organisations also contribute by providing feedback on how the student integrated into the service and addressed community needs, and the overall success of the placement. Post-placement meetings and surveys are used to identify challenges and inform adjustments for future role-emerging placements, ensuring continuous improvement in the design and delivery of these placements (Lau et al., 2019). This evaluation process fosters ongoing collaboration between educational institutions, students and host organisations, ensuring that role-emerging placements remain relevant, impactful, and aligned with both educational and community needs (Overton et al., 2009).

PRACTICE EXAMPLES

Practice example 1: occupational therapy at GCU

Whilst models of role-emerging placements may have changed over time, these have been integral to occupational therapy education at GCU since 1995. As the university for the Common Good, GCU's core values of integrity, confidence, creativity and responsibility underpin the Common Good attributes of *active and global citizenship*, *entrepreneurial mind-set*, *responsible leadership*, *systems thinking*, *confidence*, *resilience*, *compassion* and *empathy*. Students on role-emerging placements utilise their learning about asset-based approaches and social entrepreneurialism to address needs of communities whilst developing and demonstrating GCU values and attributes, introducing occupational therapy values into new settings.

GCU's current occupational therapy role-emerging placement sees third-year undergraduate and second-year MSc pre-registration students allocated to a service in pairs, part time for seven weeks. Students have pre-placement preparation including learning about asset-based approaches and social entrepreneurialism, a recap on identifying needs, a practical refresher on the core skill of activity analysis and importantly guidelines on the expectations of students, practice educators and module tutors. Assessment preparation for both assessment components is also completed pre-placement: the placement report, assessed by their practice educators, and the viva voce, which they will complete post-placement. Learning outcomes on this placement include demonstrating professional behaviour; analysing practice and behaviour commensurate with professional and regulatory body standards; analysing how the organisation meets needs of the community; analysing the use of asset-based approaches in facilitating participation, health and wellbeing; analysing and demonstrating ability to select, plan, implement and evaluate occupation focused practice; and analysing the concept of social entrepreneurialism in relation to occupational therapy and/or occupational science. A key objective of this placement is to plan, deliver and evaluate two occupation-focused interventions using an asset-based approach to address identified needs, facilitating participation, health and wellbeing. All role-emerging practice educators are invited to an information session prior to placement to communicate key information and discuss mutual expectations. Students are guided though their placement by weekly workbook activities which include on-site and directed learning activities, engaging with which supports successful completion of placement and preparation for their viva voce. Supervision during placement is twofold: student pairs/small groups receive weekly on-site supervision with their practice educator and weekly group supervision on campus with two lecturers, who are registered occupational therapists. Students maintain supervision records for both weekly supervisions as part of their placement portfolio. Following placement, students attend a post-placement session where they reflect on their key learning from placement, for example in relation to professional skills developed, how their understanding of the profession has evolved and how they may have developed personally and academically. Students are also encouraged to reflect on their learning and demonstration of an asset-based approach and social entrepreneurialism and consider how these may inform their future practice.

Students are placed within a wide range of settings, including care homes, youth services, schools, social enterprises, vocational/employability training services, supported housing, carers' centres and grassroots community initiatives. Examples of student work has included the development of sensory gardens, walking and creative groups, and falls prevention interventions. Students have supported individuals to develop independent living skills such as budgeting and cooking, implemented handwriting skills sessions, developed games to aid learning and utilised Playlist for Life. They have also supported lifespan transitions, built networks with community partners, enhanced accessibility and inclusive use of spaces, and enhanced participation in various individual and group-based meaningful activities.

The impact of role-emerging placements is beautifully illustrated through one service which has hosted GCU occupational therapy students for several years and students from another Scottish university. The service recognised the value and contribution of student occupational therapists and consequently created a new post to recruit an experienced occupational therapist. The CEO of another service – a social enterprise which frequently hosts GCU role-emerging placements – was keen to highlight some of our students' work to other organisations to demonstrate the benefits of hosting occupational therapy students. Feedback from our role-emerging partners is highly positive, recognising our students as enthusiastic and innovative. A service which runs community groups for older adults has found that the role-emerging placement benefits them in several ways, commenting that it brings out the best in the service users and that interventions leave a legacy, having introduced innovative ideas for activities that become part of weekly sessions. They have found that having students makes them consider their daily work from a fresh perspective. Having occupational therapy students from Scottish universities has prompted the CEO to want to pursue further joint work with the occupational therapy profession.

In addition to having a positive impact on services and service users, students report benefits from their role-emerging placement immediately after placement, on reflection towards the end of the programme and once they are out in practice. On return from placement, students have reported valuing the increased autonomy and the opportunity to be creative and overcome challenges, develop their knowledge and the opportunity for teamwork and building resilience. Students approaching the end of the programme have reflected on their role-emerging placement, stating it provided opportunities to really develop their observation, active listening, creativity, activity analysis, problem solving and confidence in their reasoning. A greater understanding of the importance of assets, particularly of service users, and how to support individuals and communities to identify and use these has been reported as another particular advantage of the role-emerging placement. Occupational therapists in practice have also reflected on their role-emerging placement at GCU, recounting that it taught them about group work, responsibility and communication, and developed their confidence in effectively applying theory to practice without direct supervision, all of which supported a successful final placement and transition to practice.

In undertaking a role-emerging placement, GCU students embody the Common Good ethos, develop their occupational therapy and transferable skills, and have a positive impact on communities.

Practice example 2: dietetics in schools pilot project – GCU, Scotland, UK

PrBL within dietetics in Scotland currently has a strong clinical focus, with current providers exclusively NHS Health boards across Scotland. The British Dietetic Association (BDA) (2023, p. 10) states that PrBL "may take place and is encouraged to do so in both clinical and non-clinical settings". The British Dietetic Association further describe role-emerging PrBL as "Where a learner is placed within an organisation, or an area of service, where there is currently no dietitian employed". Organisations include care homes, charity organisations and across Public Health; however, within Scotland, dietetic learners do not routinely undertake PrBL within such settings. However, higher education institutions across Scotland offering dietetic programmes have begun with identifying novel PrBL approaches to alleviate pressure on NHS departments. The development and subsequent integration of high-quality and innovative PrBL opportunities may expand learner capacity across higher education institution dietetic programmes whilst providing learners with diverse training experiences to optimise post-registration employment.

Lecturers within the Nutrition and Dietetic Department at GCU led a pilot project which aimed to test a novel PrBL model. On review of various settings, the education sector was selected in which to conduct the pilot. The education setting offers a wide range of learning and development opportunities for dietetic learners, outlined in Table 8.2.

Planning the placement model was challenging. Learning outcomes were mapped to opportunities available within the school, with additional clinical time identified

Table 8.2 Potential development opportunities with education

Application of knowledge and skills	Skill development
• Community initiatives and education: food pantries, cooling classes, cooking on a budget, menu planning, food hygiene. • Assisting with school menu planning/healthy snacks, contributing to new ideas and evaluation of current service, cost analysis. • Promoting sustainability. • Curriculum development: lesson planning and assisting delivery. • Health promotion: nutrition and lifestyle education. • Promoting healthy communities: asset mapping, working with home-school link work, health and wellbeing teams.	• Demonstrate dietetic knowledge, values, behaviour and skills. • Responsibility and creativity. • Interprofessional working. • Professional behaviour. • Effective communication skills. • Quality improvement and evaluation. • Independent practice. • Community exposure-promoting compassionate client/service user care. • Reflection and critical appraisal of practice. • Raise profile of dietetic profession and public health role of dietitians and allied health professionals.

as a need. A standard portfolio with a clinical focus was utilised to evidence competency and avoid any challenges for learners on future placements. Long-arm supervision was drawn from a dietitian working in a non-traditional NHS setting, as well as faculty staff. The placement was also interprofessional, with the pairing of dietetics and occupational therapy students.

Skills and knowledge gained on the role-emerging placement pilot as reported by learners were the following.

- Knowledge about how to interact with children/young people.
- Improved content and layout in workshops for children/young people.
- Explaining nutritional information in a straightforward way.
- Vast experience when presenting for audiences.
- To be able to increase the amount of work and complete clinical reasoning under pressure.
- Soft skills and how to approach patients, relevant skills for a dietitian.

During the pilot, certain challenges were encountered in both the planning and throughout the placement, including, for example, learner transport issues, workshop content delivery within the school and evidence collation for the portfolio element. Issues were resolved by joint meetings with higher education institution staff, learners and practice educators. Conducting a needs assessment within the host organisation and timetabling set activities in advance may provide greater placement structure and focus. Practice educators in both settings met regularly with the learner; meetings with the higher education institution link were on an as requested basis, but it may be beneficial to arrange regular set meetings for continuity.

The pilot demonstrated that learning outcomes can be met through a role-emerging PrBL model. Further collaboration and agreement amongst stakeholders are required to facilitate the incorporation of role-emerging, innovative PrBL across dietetics in Scotland. Increasing placement diversity will support diverse roles within the dietetic workforce and contribute to overall workforce sustainability (Graham and Volkert, 2022).

SUMMING UP

Role-emerging placements offer an innovative, transformative learning experience that prepares students for future healthcare challenges while expanding the reach of allied health professions. Through strategic partnerships, structured supervision, student preparation, clear learning objectives and strong assessment models, universities can ensure that role-emerging placements provide a rich, dynamic and impactful learning journey. By addressing challenges proactively and fostering collaborative, interprofessional and community-based learning, role-emerging placements not only enhance student competencies but also drive meaningful change in underserved populations and healthcare settings.

REFERENCES

BDA. (2023). *Pre-registration dietetic practice-based learning guidance*. BDA England UK, p. 10. Available at: https://www.bda.uk.com/static/c20607b6-6f03-4b58-82ab10a2dbc3b554/Pre-registration-Dietetic-PBL-Guidance-v3.pdf

Bossers, A., Cook, J., Polatajko, H. and Laine, C. (1997). Understanding the role-emerging fieldwork placement. *Canadian Journal of Occupational Therapy*, *64*(1), pp. 70–81.

Clarke, C., de Visser, R. and Sadlo, G. (2014). Role-emerging placements: A useful model for occupational therapy practice education? A review of the literature. *International Journal of Practice-Based Learning in Health and Social Care*, *2*(2), pp. 14–26.

Clarke, C., de Visser, R. and Sadlo, G. (2019). From trepidation to transformation: Strategies used by occupational therapy students on role-emerging placements. *International Journal of Practice-Based Learning in Health and Social Care*, *7*(1), pp. 18–31. https://doi.org/10.18552/ijpblhsc.v7i1.508

Clarke, C., Martin, M., de Visser, R. and Sadlo, G. (2015a). Sustaining professional identity in practice following role-emerging placements: Opportunities and challenges for occupational therapists. *British Journal of Occupational Therapy*, *78*(1), pp. 42–50. https://doi.org/10.1177/0308022614561238

Clarke, C., Martin, M., Sadlo, G. and de Visser, R. (2015b). "Facing uncharted waters": Challenges experienced by occupational therapy students undertaking role-emerging placements. *International Journal of Practice-Based Learning in Health and Social Care*, *3*(1), pp. 30–45.

Cooper, R. and Raine, R. (2009). Exploring the effect of role-emerging placements on student's professional identity. *British Journal of Occupational Therapy*, *72*(7), pp. 302–310.

Dancza, K., Warren, A., Copley, J., Rodger, S., Moran, M., McKay, E. and Taylor, A. (2013, December). Learning experiences on role-emerging placements: An exploration from the students' perspective. *Australian Occupational Therapy Journal*, *60*(6), pp. 427–435. https://doi.org/10.1111/1440-1630.12079. Epub 2013 September 1. PMID: 24299482.

Deaves, A., Matson, R., Rushe, E., et al. (2024). Exploring alternative practice placement models in occupational therapy and physiotherapy: Perspectives and experiences of learners and practice educators: A qualitative systematic review. *BMC Medical Education*, *24*, p. 1325. https://doi.org/10.1186/s12909-024-06323-z

Graham, A. and Volkert, A. (2022, February). Our students are off to school. In *Dietetics: Membership Magazine of the British Dietetics Association*. London: British Dietetic Association.

Kyte, R., Frank, H. and Thomas, Y. (2018). Physiotherapy students' experiences of role emerging placements; a qualitative study. *International Journal of Practice-Based Learning in Health and Social Care*, *6*(2), pp. 1–13.

Lau, M. and Ravenek, M. (2019). The student perspective on role-emerging fieldwork placements in cccupational therapy: A review of the literature. *The Open Journal of Occupational Therapy*, *7*(3), pp. 1–21. https://doi.org/10.15453/2168-6408.1544

Mattila, A., Deluliis, E. D. and Cook, A. B. (2018). Increasing self-efficacy through role emerging placements: Implications for occupational therapy experiential learning. *Journal of Occupational Therapy Education*, *2*(3), p. 3.

Overton, A., Clark, M. and Thomas, Y. (2009). A review of non-traditional occupational therapy practice placement education: A focus on role-emerging and project placements. *British Journal of Occupational Therapy*, *72*(7), pp. 294–301.

Rodger, S., Fitzgerald, C., Davila, W., Millar, F. and Allison, H. (2009). What makes a quality occupational therapy practice placement?" *Australian Occupational Therapy Journal*, *57*(6), pp. 371–378.

Syed, S. and Duncan, A. (2019). Role emerging placements: Skills development, postgraduate employment, and career pathways. *The Open Journal of Occupational Therapy*, *7*(1). https://doi.org/10.15453/2168-6408.1489

Thew, M., Edwards, M., Baptiste, S. and Molineux, M. (2011). *Role Emerging Occupational Therapy: Maximising Occupation-Focused Practice*. Chichester: Wiley-Blackwell.

Thew, M., Hargreaves, A. and Cronin-Davis, J. (2008). An evaluation of role-emerging practice placement model for a full cohort of occupational therapy students. *British Journal of Occupational Therapy*, *71*(8), pp. 348–353.

Thew, M., Thomas, Y. and Briggs, M. (2018, June). The impact of a role emerging placement while a student occupational therapist, on subsequent qualified employability, practice, and career path. *Australian Occupational Therapy Journal*, *65*(3), pp. 198–207. https://doi.org/10.1111/1440-1630.12463. Epub 2018 March 11. PMID: 29527692.

Think Pacific. (n.d.). *Remote internships – Fiji Islands: How does it work*? Available at: Remote internships | Fiji Islands | Think Pacific. (Accessed 24 March 2025).

Thomas, Y. and Rodger, S. (2011). Successful role emerging placements: It is all in the preparation. In M. Thew, M. Edwards, S. Baptiste and M. Molineux (Eds.), *Role Emerging Occupational Therapy* (pp. 39–53). Chichester: Wiley-Blackwell.

Warren, A. F. (2014). *Innovation, personal growth, and professional identity: Perspectives on role emerging placements in occupational therapy*. Available at: https://hdl.handle.net/10344/3996 (Accessed 24 March 2025).

Chapter 9
Interprofessional placements

Pragashnie Govender and Deshini Naidoo

CHAPTER OVERVIEW

Interprofessional education (IPE) is a cornerstone of modern healthcare training, fostering collaboration among professionals to improve patient care and safety. This chapter explores the significance of IPE and its practical application through interprofessional placements, which provide immersive, real-world learning experiences for students across healthcare disciplines. Traditional classroom-based IPE lays the foundation for interprofessional competencies, but IPP enhances these skills through hands-on engagement in clinical and community settings. The chapter examines key considerations for designing and implementing effective IPP placements, including organisational structures, curriculum alignment, competency development and interprofessional supervision. Challenges such as resource allocation, scheduling conflicts and institutional attitudes toward IPE are also discussed. Additionally, the chapter highlights various educational strategies, including simulation-based learning, case discussions and peer-assisted learning, which contribute to the development of interprofessional competencies. The chapter underscores the broader impact of IPP, emphasising its role in enhancing professional identity formation, fostering mutual respect among disciplines and ultimately improving healthcare delivery. By addressing the complexities of interprofessional collaboration, this chapter provides a comprehensive guide to integrating IPP into allied healthcare education for a more cohesive and patient-centred approach to care.

CHAPTER OBJECTIVES

The objectives of this chapter are the following.

- To present an overview of interprofessional placement for health professions education.

DOI: 10.4324/9781003411765-9

- To describe design features for models of interprofessional placements for health professions.
- To present fundamental principles derived from the evidence and to provide a case example for interprofessional placements.

INTRODUCTION

IPE is foundational to advancing collaborative healthcare practice, ultimately enhancing the quality of patient care and ensuring patient safety. IPE involves educational experiences whereby students from two or more healthcare professions learn with, from and about each other to improve practice. This interaction provides ideal opportunities to develop interprofessional competencies that directly translate into collaborative practice,[1] whereby comprehensive services are delivered by a team of healthcare professionals from diverse backgrounds. Collaborative practice is particularly impactful, as it brings together varied perspectives and areas of expertise, allowing these professionals to work with patients and their families, carers and communities to ensure the delivery of high-quality care in a range of settings (Mattiazzi et al., 2023a). Such collaborative approaches are integral in responding to today's complex healthcare challenges and meeting diverse patient needs through coordinated, efficient and effective care delivery.

The importance of incorporating IPE within health professions education is widely recognised, as it plays a critical role in preparing healthcare providers to work collaboratively with others, creating a less hierarchical and more inclusive environment. IPE and curriculum elements like interprofessional placements are essential in equipping practitioners of the 21st century with the skills needed to collaborate effectively with a broad range of stakeholders. As argued by Bhutta et al. (2010) and Frenk et al. (2010), healthcare education must adapt to encourage less hierarchical, cross-disciplinary partnerships to foster a more holistic approach to patient care.

Traditionally, IPE has been delivered in campus- or classroom-based settings. This approach has been largely effective in reaching a large cohort of students and

---

1   When members of more than one health or social care (or both) profession learn interactively together, for the explicit purpose of improving interprofessional collaboration or the health/wellbeing (or both) of patients/clients (Reeves et al., 2013).

providing foundational knowledge for collaborative practice. Classroom-based IPE formats are advantageous in terms of scalability, as they can accommodate many students, offer structured environments and can be efficiently integrated into academic schedules (Lapkin et al., 2013). However, classroom settings may lack the practical, hands-on experiences that are crucial for truly effective interprofessional learning. Practice-based learning experiences, particularly through IPP, offer more engaging and practical settings for students to strengthen their collaborative competencies. Research indicates that these placements can be highly effective in reinforcing interprofessional skills and providing a more relevant, motivating educational experience for students (Aggar et al., 2020).

IPP serves as the bridge between theoretical, classroom-based IPE and practical, real-world application. IPP follows a continuum that spans multiple training levels, beginning with preparatory learning through various educational strategies and culminating in active, immersive learning experiences. This continuum allows students to build foundational skills before applying them in clinical settings, where they interact with actual patients and professionals from other fields. This structured progression and interactive learning[2] through training levels ensures that students are well-prepared and can gain the most from their placement experiences (Kaas-Mason et al., 2024). IPP commonly takes place in settings such as interprofessional training wards, student-led clinics, community health centres, hospitals, home visiting services, outpatient clinics, primary care centres and community service learning locations. Additional venues include screening clinics, community events and nursing homes (Mattiazzi et al., 2023a). Each of these environments offers unique opportunities for students to engage in collaborative practice, apply interprofessional skills and gain a more comprehensive understanding of patient-centred care. In these settings, students work directly with patients, often in high-pressure, real-life situations, which encourages the development of critical competencies required for successful interprofessional practice. Universities are also positioned to address societal needs through integrated service provision offered via IPP.

The benefits of IPP extend beyond individual student outcomes, promoting patient safety and improving care quality. In a systematic review, Mattiazzi et al. (2023a) found that most studies reported positive outcomes resulting from IPE interventions in clinical training for health professional students. Immersive IPP experiences foster teamwork, communication and a deeper

---

2 Interactive learning requires active learner participation and active exchange between learners from different professions (Reeves et al., 2013, p. 4).

understanding of professional roles and boundaries, which in turn leads to respect for other professions and clarity on professional scope of practice. Moreover, by learning to adopt the patient's perspective, students develop a deeper sense of empathy and commitment to patient-centred care, facilitating better relationships and communication among healthcare providers (Mattiazzi et al., 2023a; Malone et al., 2022).

In summary, IPP plays an essential role in bridging academic learning with practical skills, helping students to gain confidence, competence and the essential collaborative abilities needed in today's healthcare landscape. It supports the development of professional identities and fosters the skills, attitudes and knowledge needed for students to navigate interprofessional boundaries and work collaboratively with other healthcare providers.

CONSIDERATIONS FOR DESIGNING IPP PLACEMENT

For effective IPP implementation, several considerations are required. These include – but are not limited to – the organisational structure and culture, available resources, practice protocols, having a common language, how teaching and learning can be linked with intended learning outcomes and assessment, trained facilitators and availability of funding for implementation (Mattiazzi et al., 2023b; Martin and Sy, 2021; Reeves et al., 2013). There are several potential challenges in implementing an IPP that need to be taken into consideration. These include finding shared time and coordinating differing numbers of students from different professions into interprofessional teams for the placement (Salfi et al., 2012; Thistlethwaite, 2015). Additionally, the availability of sufficient funding, time allocation and having an adequate number of student placements for the placement need to be considered when planning the IPP (Reeves and Hean, 2013). The institutional culture and the attitude of the students and the educators toward the IPP are also to be explored. If students or educators feel unprepared or have negative attitudes, the success of the IPP may be jeopardised (Liston et al., 2011).

Crossing boundaries

Interprofessional learning among students from various professions during their clinical placements can be a complex process. The structure of settings and the diverse group of healthcare professionals necessitate a team-based approach to enhance care (Smith et al., 2018). To facilitate this learning, it may be necessary to assist students in navigating the boundaries between different professions (Figure 9.1). Interprofessional practice involves interacting and negotiating across

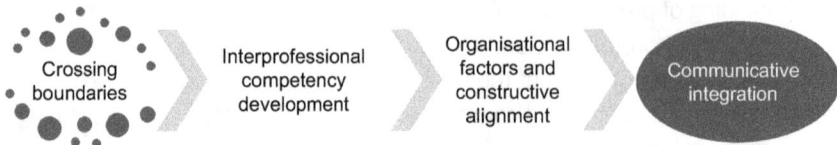

Figure 9.1 Crossing boundaries to support IPP placements

these boundaries. The mechanisms proposed to promote this boundary-crossing learning and interprofessional development include identification, coordination, reflection and transformation (Bivall et al., 2021). Students should be encouraged to identify similarities and differences in their professional roles towards achieving a shared understanding and respectful acceptance. Effective coordination involves developing clear communication to collaborate across professional boundaries while maintaining unity. As students become reflective practitioners, they should acknowledge differences between their own practices and those of their team members. Shared experiences can enhance understanding and appreciation across different professions. Students should have opportunities to transform their understanding of teamwork by modifying existing practices or redefining their approach (Bivall et al., 2021; Bakker and Akkerman, 2019). These mechanisms offer valuable approaches to explore and comprehend the intricacies of interprofessional learning among students from diverse professions during their IPP.

Interprofessional competency development

In interprofessional competency development during IPP, we can draw from existing interprofessional competency frameworks, such as the Interprofessional Education Collaborative (IPEC 2023). Notwithstanding this, a one-size-fits-all approach has limitations, especially regarding the complexity of placement settings (McClaney et al., 2022). The espousal of individually defined competencies assumes that if each healthcare professional possesses and applies these competencies, it will lead to optimal interprofessional collaboration and team performance (Shinners and Franqueiro, 2017). However, delivering ideal care within an effective interprofessional team requires the collective efforts of team members (Smith et al., 2018; Langlois, 2020).

The core competencies for IPE can be summarised as including roles and responsibilities/role clarification, interprofessional values and ethical practice, interprofessional conflict resolution, communication, collaboration and teamwork, reflection and shared decision-making (McClaney et al., 2022; van Diggele et al.,

2020; IPEC, 2023). One or more of these competencies should be considered as an outcome when designing an interprofessional activity and, where possible, matched to an assessment task.

Organisational factors and alignment to learning outcomes and assessment

Organisational support is critical to facilitating shared space on the timetable and for logistic support (Reeves et al., 2013; 2007). Team meetings, workshops and negotiations between the clinical site and the higher education institution are required to ensure mutual goals for the placements and agreements on the IPE activities in which the students would engage and how to facilitate the most conducive learning environments (Mattiazzi et al., 2023b). There is a need for the IPP to be integrated into the curriculum for the students to acknowledge the relevance of the placement and to ensure the timing of the placement is appropriate (Doucet et al., 2014; Reeves et al., 2013). Curriculum developers are required to consider several factors, including creating opportunities for IPE exposure for each cohort across each level of study and scaffolding to allow students opportunities to use their knowledge and skills in a safe space (simulations, case-based discussions, etc.). Additionally, there needs to be constructive alignment between the intended learning outcomes for the placements, the teaching and learning strategies used, and the assessment of the students for placement to be of relevance to the students (Doucet et al., 2014). These may prepare students to navigate IPP complexities in a clinical setting.

Communicative integration and the use of operative models in an IPE context

The International Classification of Functioning, Disability and Health (ICF) and the community-based rehabilitation (CBR) matrix, both developed by the World Health Organization, are frameworks that facilitate interprofessional practice for individuals and in the community (Rhoda et al., 2016). IPP activities allow students to familiarise themselves with the different languages and tasks of each other's professions. The ICF has been proposed as a common language that facilitates shared assessment and goal setting between students of various health professions (Friedman and Nealon, 2023). Using theory or a framework can assist in providing a common understanding of the intended goals for client intervention and practical solutions to issues that arise during the placement, as well as providing the justification for inclusion of IPP (Reeves and Hean, 2013; Hean et al.,

2009). Some practical methods to apply IPE theory during the placement include using the ICF to formulate simulation-based learning or case discussions (Soubra et al., 2018).

Approach to supervision and IPP facilitation

Facilitating interprofessional groups of students in a clinical setting requires a distinct skill set that combines confidence, adaptability in managing professional conflicts and a strong commitment to IPE. This process begins with educators upskilling in this area, enabling them to facilitate evidence-informed and intentional interprofessional practice (Egan-Lee et al., 2011). Effective mentorship or facilitation should be carried out by trained professionals with expertise in a specific field or a related profession, ensuring that students receive relevant and applicable feedback. Throughout the placement, mentors and facilitators play a crucial role in guiding students, fostering collaboration and helping them develop the skills necessary for effective teamwork in their professional practice.

Mode of delivery in IPP

From an educational perspective, interprofessional learning in the workplace is typically structured around various activities integrated into clinical placements. These familiar and widely used educational approaches include patient interviews, case studies, case discussions, case-based learning, structured workshops, ward rounds, shadowing, observations, seminars, student-led clinics, student teams and simulation-based learning. Additionally, initiatives such as Schwartz Rounds, joint client sessions, home-based care and writing or reviewing healthcare team notes and records further enhance collaborative learning. Community mentors or individuals attending student discussions in university or clinical settings also contribute valuable insights. These learning experiences can take various forms, including in-person contact-based interactions, telehealth-based education and blended learning approaches that combine both virtual and face-to-face engagement.

Planning and preparation for IPP

Establishing a successful interprofessional practice begins with identifying key competencies and aligning them with the intended learning outcomes. This process includes selecting appropriate frameworks and approaches to IPE within the IPP, ensuring that the structure supports meaningful collaboration. Additionally, it is crucial to assess resource needs, logistical requirements and the availability of suitable spaces for effective interprofessional practice. Engaging stakeholders through consultation fosters strong relationships and helps in defining shared goals for the programme (Baerheim and Raaheim, 2019; Laing and Bacevice, 2013). Training staff and facilitators is essential to ensure they are equipped to guide students effectively. Moreover, selecting appropriate educational strategies and aligning them with assessment methods strengthens the learning experience. Consideration must also be given to the frequency and duration of supervision, as well as the facilitation model that will best support student development in an interprofessional setting.

Implementing IPP

In an interprofessional learning environment, students are exposed to the complexities of daily practice and the challenges that professionals face in collaborative healthcare settings, including the diverse modes of interprofessional collaboration (Reeves et al., 2018). Facilitators play a critical role in navigating the intricate relationship between individual professional responsibilities and team dynamics (Lingard et al., 2017). They must also be mindful of power structures and stereotypes that can influence collaboration and take steps to address these challenges (Nancarrow et al., 2013).

Supervision and facilitation require ongoing monitoring and evaluation to ensure effectiveness, as interprofessional learning does not occur automatically simply by bringing different professionals together. Instead, it must be deliberately guided to foster meaningful collaboration. A psychologically safe learning environment is essential, allowing students from all professions to engage confidently in teamwork and skill development (Maddock et al., 2023).

Providing ample opportunities for students to participate in ward rounds, team meetings, combined projects, case-based discussions, on-site case management and student-led clinics is crucial in reinforcing their learning experience. Additionally, structured facilitation should support synchronous patient consultations, the collaborative development of integrative healthcare plans beyond patient interactions and engagement in professional socialisation within healthcare teams (Mattiazzi et al., 2023a).

PAL provides students with valuable opportunities to observe, share experiences and learn – both within their own profession and in collaboration with others. This approach not only enhances their understanding of different professional roles and scopes but also positively influences the development of their professional identity (van Diggele et al., 2020). Within interprofessional practice, PAL can be facilitated directly, such as through structured tutorials, or indirectly, such as through peer observation and feedback in clinical settings. Allocating protected time for PAL allows senior students to support junior learners, fostering a supportive learning environment. Additionally, peer observation and debriefing create a non-threatening space for students to reflect and enhance their learning (Prince et al., 2010). The co-location of student workspaces further encourages informal and indirect peer-assisted learning, facilitating spontaneous collaboration and knowledge sharing among students (Martin and Sy, 2021).

Post-placement consideration for IPP

Reflection and debriefing following a placement are crucial in helping students critically assess their experiences, identify what was effective and consider how they can improve their approach in future interprofessional encounters (Reeves et al., 2007). Additionally, a thorough review and evaluation of the IPP placement (Table 9.1), including the supervisory model and overall structure, can provide valuable insights to enhance future IPP initiatives and optimise outcomes. Constructive feedback from students, facilitators and stakeholders plays a key role in refining the learning experience and ensuring continuous improvement in IPE and practice.

PRACTICE EXAMPLES OF IPP

BOX 9.1   CASE EXAMPLE FROM SOUTH AFRICA OF TWO IPP MODULES

Level 1 Community Studies module

This an interprofessional first-year module designed to facilitate students' understanding of the community, primary healthcare, the roles and responsibilities of different professions, and planning goals with the community members. The students include dental therapy and oral health, occupational therapy, audiology, speech, language therapy and biokinetics, and exercise and leisure science.

This module introduces students to the concept of interprofessional work that they will engage in the community in the final year of their degrees. The students complete didactic sessions that outline the basic concepts around interprofessional practice, what different professions do and their roles in healthcare, primary healthcare, and introduction to community entry. The students complete the didactic session in interdisciplinary groups and conduct five structured visits to the community, learning how to interview community members in their contextual environment. The students use logs to reflect on their understanding of community engagement and how the interprofessional team can work together. Additionally, as part of their assessment, the interprofessional student groups plan how to implement a health promotion campaign in their assigned community.

Level 4 Community Studies module

In their final year, occupational therapy, audiology, speech and language therapy, and optometry students are embedded in an under-resourced local community. Each programme has a credit-bearing community module to provide community-based learning experiences for final-year students. The modules are standalone modules that last either a semester or across the year. The students must visit families as part of an interdisciplinary team and provide services at a local primary healthcare clinic. Additionally, the students conduct health promotion programmes at the local schools. The interdisciplinary team has to meet at least once a week. At the end of the course, the students must present a joint oral case presentation on a client they have been providing services for and a joint project that would assist the community. Examples of these projects include an innovative to sell used clothing as income generation project to empower women in the community, an early childhood development programme for the local school for children aged 4–5 years, a gardening project for income generation, etc.

Key learning outcomes

1. To enhance the student's understanding of each other's roles and how the team could approach clinical and social problems.
2. To promote the students' ability to consult and refer to other team members when the client's issue is beyond the students' scope of practice.
3. To facilitate collaboration effectively with others to assess, plan, provide and review care that promotes health outcomes for patients.
4. To promote effective teamwork with other health professionals in a variety of venues and practice settings.
5. To promote the development of consensus building and appropriate nego-tiation/conflict management skills when resolving issues and concerns in a team.

Table 9.1 Design principles for interprofessional placement

Approach to supervision/ IPP facilitation	Facilitators of interprofessional groups of students in the clinical setting requires a specific skill set, incorporating a range of attributes (confidence, flexibility in managing professional conflict and a commitment to IPE) and begins with the educator first upskilling in this area (Egan-Lee et al., 2011), which helps with facilitating an evidence-informed and intentional IPP.
	Mentorship or facilitation needs to be conducted by trained mentors/facilitators. Facilitators or mentors need to be professional specific or a profession with similar focus so that the students can gain relevant feedback that can be used in their profession.
	Mentors/facilitators during the placement facilitate the group and guide students on how to work collaboratively.
Mode of delivery	From an educational standpoint, interprofessional learning among students in the workplace has been structured as activities during clinical placements. These arrangements are familiar and commonly used in educational settings. These include patient interviews, case studies, case discussions, case-based learning, structured workshops, ward rounds, shadowing, observations, seminars, student-led clinics, student teams, simulation-based learning, Schwartz Rounds, joint client sessions, home-based care, writing and reviewing healthcare team notes and records, and community mentors/persons who attend student discussions at the university/clinical setting.
	Contact-based, telehealth, blended learning.
Planning and preparation	Identifying competencies and linking these to the intended learning outcomes of the IPP.
	Decision on frameworks and approaches to IPE within the IPP.
	Identification of resource needs, logistical supports and available spaces for collaborative interprofessional practice.
	Stakeholder identification and consultation are needed to develop relationships to develop clearly framed common goals for the IPP (Baerheim and Raaheim, 2019; Laing and Bacevice, 2013).
	Training of staff and facilitators within the IPP.
	Identification of educational strategies for IPP and alignment to assessment and assessment.
	Consider frequency and duration of supervision/facilitation.
	Consider the supervisory/facilitation model that is to be adopted.

Implementing placement	In this context, students encounter the intricacy of daily work and the challenges practitioners deal with in relation to interprofessional collaboration, such as a multitude of interprofessional modes of collaboration (Reeves et al., 2018). Facilitators must navigate the complex relationship between the professional and the team/group dynamics (Lingard et al., 2017). Being aware of and managing issues of power structures and stereotypes (Nancarrow et al., 2013). Monitor and evaluate the frequency and duration of supervision/facilitation. Interprofessional learning must be facilitated and cannot be assumed to occur naturally by merely gathering different professionals. Students from all included professions require a learning environment where their psychological safety is assured (Maddock et al., 2023). Students should feel safe to collaborate or practice skills (Maddock et al., 2023). Ensuring that students have sufficient opportunity to engage in ward rounds team meetings, combined projects, case-based discussions, case management on site, student-led clinics, etc. Facilitation of synchronous patient consultations, collaborative development of integrative healthcare plans outside of patient consultations and participation in socialisation with healthcare teams (Mattiazzi et al., 2023a).
Peer-assisted learning	PAL allows students to observe, share their experiences and learn within their own profession and with other professionals. PAL can positively influence the development of students' professional identity and their insight into professional roles and scope (van Diggele et al., 2020). During IPP, PAL can be facilitated either directly via tutorials, for example, or indirectly, for example by peer observation and feedback on the ward. Students can be provided with protected time to engage in PAL, whereas a more senior student can assist more junior learners in the IPP. Peer observation and debriefing offer a non-threatening opportunity to promote learning (Prince et al., 2010). Co-location of student workspaces can facilitate indirect/informal peer-assisted learning among students (Martin and Sy, 2021).
Post-placement	Reflection and debriefing after the placement are essential to facilitate students' reasoning on what worked and how it could have been done better for future encounters (Reeves et al., 2007). Review and evaluate of the IPP placement, supervisory model and structure of placement to influence future IPP and for optimal outcomes. Solicit feedback to improve future IPP initiatives.

KEY PRINCIPLES OF IPP

Effective IPP is grounded in strategic planning and thoughtful implementation, integrating interprofessional competencies into learning outcomes while ensuring appropriate resources and fostering stakeholder collaboration. Facilitators are central to this process, guiding students' reflection, nurturing understanding and skilfully managing group dynamics to balance support with student autonomy. Through IPP, students develop professional identities and competencies, building mutual respect, clinical confidence and enhanced problem-solving skills within diverse teams. Carefully designed activities, including reflection and peer learning, promote joint decision-making and client-centred care, equipping students for effective, collaborative practice in real-world healthcare settings.

IPP requires careful planning and implementation to facilitate successful learning outcomes

1. Integration of the interprofessional practice competencies into the intended learning outcomes of the IPP, including use of a common language.
2. Consideration of the logistics, infrastructure and resources for shared spaces for interprofessional practice (Reeves et al., 2013).
3. Engagement with stakeholders to develop relationships, understand organisational culture and develop shared goals for the IPP.
4. Constructively align educational strategies with IPP and assessment (Doucet et al., 2014).

IPP facilitators are required to ensure successful outcomes

1. Facilitating the development of student insight and subsequent translation of learning to practice (Maddock et al., 2023; van Diggele et al., 2020).
2. Guiding the debriefing, provoking individual thought and engaging participants to make sense of theory and simulation concepts in practice (Maddock et al., 2023; van Diggele et al., 2020).
3. Being conscious of professional stereotypes and the importance of allowing students time to solve problems together and interact in a safe setting (Maddock et al., 2023; van Diggele et al., 2020).
4. Assisting in mediating group dynamics and conflict resolution (Maddock et al., 2023; van Diggele et al., 2020; IPEC, 2023).
5. Facilitating an appropriate balance between facilitator support and student autonomy.
6. Clarifying role blurring, confusion over boundaries and responsibilities (IPEC, 2023).

7. Workplace modelling to teach affective competencies (Maddock et al., 2023; van Diggele et al., 2020).

IPP assists in the development of professional identity and competencies

1. Fosters understanding of different professional roles and the patient's viewpoint (Kent and Keating, 2015; IPEC, 2023).
2. Through effective communication and enhanced relationships with one another and develop shared normative outlooks (Aggar et al., 2020; IPEC, 2023).
3. Promotes positive attitudes and respect towards other professions and opportunities for exploring professional identities (Reeves et al., 2018; Aggar et al., 2020).
4. Improved confidence with clinical skills and confidence in interacting with students from other disciplines (Kent and Keating, 2015; Aggar et al., 2020).
5. Developing stronger problem-solving skills due to their interprofessional teamwork opportunities and valuing joint decision-making (Lapkin et al., 2013; Aggar et al., 2020; IPEC, 2023).

Careful selection of activities to promote effective IPP and attainment of competencies

1. Activities used during IPP need to promote interprofessional teamwork and identity (Martin and Sy, 2021; Mattiazzi et al., 2023a, 2023b; IPEC, 2023).
2. Activities should foster shared/joint decision-making and goal setting (Martin and Sy, 2021; Mattiazzi et al., 2023a, 2023b; IPEC, 2023).
3. Should be geared towards holistic client-centred practice (Martin and Sy, 2021; Mattiazzi et al., 2023a, 2023b).
4. Offer opportunities for joint practice and assessments (Martin and Sy, 2021; Mattiazzi et al., 2023a, 2023b).
5. Should encourage peer-assisted learning (Martin and Sy, 2021; Mattiazzi et al., 2023a, 2023b).
6. Encourage student-led projects and case discussions (Martin and Sy, 2021; Mattiazzi et al., 2023a, 2023b).

Post-placement reflection to promote professional reasoning for future encounters

1. Reflection and debriefing after the placement are essential to facilitate students' reasoning on what worked and how it could have been done better for future encounters (Reeves et al., 2007).

CONCLUSION

This chapter explores IPP as a crucial component of health professions education, aiming to cultivate collaborative practice skills for high-quality patient care. By immersing students from diverse health fields in real-world clinical settings, IPP promotes teamwork, mutual respect and an understanding of each profession's roles. Effective IPP requires strategic planning, clear learning objectives and resources such as shared spaces and trained facilitators. Placement settings range widely, from hospitals to community clinics, each providing unique opportunities for students to enhance their clinical skills, patient-centred care and collaborative problem solving. Challenges in implementation – such as scheduling, resource allocation and alignment with institutional goals – must be carefully managed. Core competencies in IPP include teamwork, communication, ethical practice and conflict resolution, which are supported through reflection, interactive learning and in application of relevant frameworks. Overall, IPP offers valuable experiential learning that builds professional identity and prepares students for integrated, effective healthcare delivery in diverse, team-oriented environments.

REFERENCES

Aggar, C., Mozolic-Staunton, B., Scorey, M., Kemp, M., Lovi, R., Lewis, S., Walker, T. and Thomas, T. (2020). Interprofessional primary healthcare student placements: Qualitative findings from a mixed-method evaluation. *International Journal of Work-Integrated Learning*, *21*(3), pp. 223–234.

Baerheim, A. and Raaheim, A. (2019). Pedagogical aspects of interprofessional workplace learning: A case study. *Journal of Interprofessional Care*, pp. 59–65.

Bakker, A. and Akkerman, S. (2019). Chapter 18. The learning potential of boundary crossing in the vocational curriculum. In D. Guile and L. Unwin (Eds.), *The Wiley Handbook of Vocational Education and Training* (pp. 349–372). Hoboken, NJ: John Wiley and Sons.

Bhutta, Z.A., Chen, L., Cohen, J., Crisp, N., Evans, T., Fineberg, H., Frenk, J., Garcia, P., Horton, R., Ke, Y., Kelley, P., Kistnasamy, B., Meleis, A., Naylor, D., Pablos-Mendez, A., Reddy, S., Scrimshaw, S., Sepulveda, J., Serwadda, D. and Zurayk, H. (2010). Education of health professionals for the 21st century: A global independent Commission. *The Lancet*, *375*(9721), p. 1137.

Bivall, A., Falk, A. and Gustavsson, M. (2021). Students' interprofessional workplace learning in clinical placement. *Professions and Professionalism*, *11*(3).

Doucet, S.A., MacKenzie, D., Loney, E., Godden-Webster, A., Lauckner, H., Brown, P.A., Andrews, C. and Packe, T.L. (2014). Curricular factors that unintentionally affect learning in a community-based interprofessional education program. *Journal of Research in Interprofessional Practice and Education*, *4*(2).

Egan-Lee, E., Baker, L., Tobin, S., Hollenberg, E., Dematteo, D. and Reeves, S. (2011). Neophyte facilitator experiences of interprofessional education: Implications for faculty development. *Journal of Interprofessional Care*, *25*, pp. 333–338.

Frenk, J., Chen, L., Bhutta, Z.A., Cohen, J., Crisp, N., Evans, T., Fineberg, H., Garcia, P., Ke, Y., Kelley, P., Kistnasamy, B., Meleis, A., Naylor, D., Pablos-Mendez, A., Reddy, S., Scrimshaw, S., Sepulveda, J., Serwadda, D. and Zurayk, H. (2010). Health professionals for a new century: Transforming education to strengthen health systems in an interdependent world. *The Lancet, 376*(9756), pp. 1923–1958.

Friedman, Z. and Nealon, K. (2023). Siloed vs. interprofessional approach: Speech language pathologists' and occupational therapists' perspectives on comorbidity of childhood apraxia of speech and sensory processing disorder. *Journal of Interprofessional Education & Practice, 31*, p. 100661.

Hean, S., Craddock, D. and O'Halloran, C. (2009). Learning theories and interprofessional education: A user's guide. *Learning in Health and Social Care, 8*(4), pp. 250–262.

IPEC. (2023). *IPEC Core Competencies for Interprofessional Collaborative Practice: Connecting Health Professions for Better Care*. Washington DC: Interprofessional Education Collaborative.

Kaas-Mason, S., Langlois, S., Bartlett, S., Friesen, F., Ng, S., Bellicoso, D. and Rowland, P. (2024). A critical interpretive synthesis of interprofessional education interventions. *Journal of Interprofessional Care*, pp. 1–10.

Kent, F. and Keating, J. (2015). Interprofessional education in primary health care for entry level students – a systematic literature review. *Nurse Education Today, 35*(12), pp. 1221–1231.

Laing, A. and Bacevice, P. (2013). Using design to drive organizational performance and innovation in the corporate workplace: Implications for interprofessional environments. *Journal of Interprofessional Care, 27*(Supplement 2), pp. 37–45.

Langlois, S. (2020). Collective competence: Moving from individual to collaborative expertise. *Perspectives in Medical Education, 9*(2), pp. 71–73.

Lapkin, S., Levett-Jones, T. and Gilligan, C. (2013). A systematic review of the effectiveness of interprofessional education in health professional programs. *Nurse Education Today, 33*(2), pp. 90–102.

Lingard, L., Sue-Chue-Lam, C., Tait, G.R., Bates, J., Shadd, J. and Schulz, V. (2017). Pulling together and pulling apart: Influences of convergence and divergence on distributed healthcare teams. *Advances in Health Science Education, 22*(5), pp. 1085–1099.

Liston, B., et al. (2011). Interprofessional education in the internal medicine clerkship: Results from a national survey. *Academic Medicine, 86*(7), pp. 872–876.

Maddock, B., Dārziņš, P. and Kent, F. (2023). Realist review of interprofessional education for health care students: What works for whom and why. *Journal of Interprofessional Care, 37*(2), pp. 173–186.

Malone, J., Hebberd, B. and Benham, A. (2022). THRIVE: A student-led, person-centred, interprofessional practice placement experience using a digital telehealth platform. Findings from a student survey. *Physiotherapy, 114*, p. e19.

Martin, P. and Sy, M. (2021). Twelve tips to facilitate Interprofessional education and collaborative practice with students on placements in healthcare settings. *The Journal of Practice Teaching and Learning, 18*(3).

Mattiazzi, J., Cottrell, N., Ng, N. and Beckman, E. (2023a). Behavioural outcomes of interprofessional education within clinical settings for health professional students: A systematic literature review. *Journal of Interprofessional Care*, pp. 1–4.

Mattiazzi, S., Cottrell, N., Ng, N. and Beckman, E. (2023b). The impact of interprofessional education interventions in health professional student clinical training: A systematic review. *Journal of Interprofessional Education & Practice, 30*(100596), pp. 1–4.

McLaney, E., Morassaei, S., Hughes, L., Davies, R., Campbell, M. and Di Prospero, L. (2022). A framework for interprofessional team collaboration in a hospital setting: Advancing team competencies and behaviours. *Healthcare Management Forum, 35*(2), pp. 112–117.

Nancarrow, S.A., Booth, A., Ariss, S., Smith, T., Enderby, P. and Roots, A. (2013). Ten principles of good interdisciplinary team work. *Human Resources for Health, 11*(19).

Prince, T., Snowden, E. and Matthews, B. (2010). Utilising peer coaching as a tool to improve student-teacher confidence and support the development of classroom practice. *Literacy Information and Computer Education Journal*, pp. 49–51.

Reeves, S., Goldman, J. and Oandasan, I. (2007). Key factors in planning and implementing interprofessional education in health care settings. *Journal of Allied Health, 36*(4), pp. 231–235.

Reeves, S. and Hean, S. (2013). Why we need theory to help us better understand the nature of interprofessional education, practice and care. *Journal of Interprofessional Care, 27*(1), pp. 1–3.

Reeves, S., Tassone, M., Parker, K., Wagner, S.J. and Simmons, B. (2013). Interprofessional education: An overview of key developments in the past three decades. *Work, 41*(3), pp. 233–245.

Reeves, S., Xyrichis, A. and Zwarenstein, M. (2018). Teamwork, collaboration, coordination, and networking: Why we need to distinguish between different types of interprofessional practice. *Journal of Interprofessional Care, 32*(1), pp. 1–3. https://doi.org/10.1080/13561820.201 7.1400150

Rhoda, A., Waggie, F., Filies, G. and Frantz, J. (2016). Using operative models (ICF and CBR) within an interprofessional context to address community needs. *African Journal of Health Professions Education, 8*(2), pp. 214–216.

Salfi, J., Solomon, P., Allen, D., Mohaupt, J. and Patterson, C. (2012). Overcoming all obstacles: A framework for embedding interprofessional education into a large, multisite Bachelor of Science Nursing program. *Journal of Nursing Education, 51*(2), p. 10.

Shinners, J. and Franqueiro, T. (2017). Individual and collective competence. *The Journal of Continuing Education in Nursing, 48*(4), pp. 148–150.

Smith, T., Fowler-Davis, S., Nancarrow, S., Ariss, S.M.B. and Enderby, P. (2018). Leadership in interprofessional health and social care teams: A literature review. *Leadership Health Services, 31*(4), pp. 452–467.

Soubra, L., Badr, S., Zahran, E. and Aboul-Seoud, M. (2018). Effect of interprofessional education on role clarification and patient care planning by health professions students. *Health Professions Education, 4*(4), pp. 317–328.

Thistlethwaite, J. (2015). Interprofessional education: Implications and development for medical education. *Educación Médica, 16*(1), pp. 68–73.

van Diggele, C., Roberts, C., Burgess, A. and Mellis, C. (2020). Interprofessional education: Tips for design and implementation. *BMC Medical Education, 20*(2), pp. 1–6.

Chapter 10

Project and research placements

Katrina Bannigan

CHAPTER OVERVIEW

Project and research placements are distinct, but closely related, placement models. This chapter provides a working definition of both models and clearly distinguishes the similarities and differences between the two. A rapid review of the literature was undertaken and the findings used, alongside experiences of facilitating these placements, to delineate the design principles of the models presented in the chapter. The key issues are choosing the project or research study itself, mapping the learning experience to the placement learning outcomes, the practice educator's approach, allowing time for planning and preparation, creating a sense of belonging, monitoring progress during the placement and using feedback to improve future placements. Practice examples are used to bring the models alive and make the link between theory and practice. Future directions for these models are considered.

CHAPTER OBJECTIVES

The objectives of this chapter are the following.

- The case for using project and research placements as models of practice-based learning.
- Working definitions of project and research placements, including how they differ from each other, and their design principles, derived from the evidence.
- Real-life case studies of project and research placements as examples of successful placements.

DOI: 10.4324/9781003411765-10

- Insight into how project and research placements can align with the wider professional aspirations of practice educators whilst also facilitating excellent learning experience for students.
- A sense of the future direction for these models of placement.

INTRODUCTION

The focus of this chapter – project and research placements as models of placement – probably creates the biggest challenge to our perceptions of what a practice placement is 'meant' to look like. In terms of practice-based learning, they are challenging because the activities on which these placements focus have been associated traditionally with learning in higher education settings. This chapter will focus on the innovation of project and research placements as models of placement rather than the wider context of traditional and non-traditional practice education (Hedley, 2023), with that said, the case for the appropriateness of project and research placements as models of practice-based learning will be outlined.

To begin, what are project and research placements? They can be university-based or conducted in health and social care services (Angus et al., 2022). A project or research study may be the placement setting or a project or study can be conducted alongside a clinical caseload as a split placement (Ashley et al., 2022). For this reason, they lend themselves to hybrid placements (see Chapter 6). There are similarities in how they are conducted; they both involve completion of, or contribution to, a practice-related project. The distinguishing feature of each is project management (project placement) and research knowledge and skills (research placement). Project placements – also referred to as "project-focused fieldwork" (Fortune et al., 2006, p. 236), a "practicum" (James et al., 2016, p. 71), "short project" placement (Thompson, 2017, p. 413) or a "project-focused model" (Beveridge and Pentland, 2020, p. 506) – centre on project management and "may focus on developing new programmes or resources, or seek to evaluate existing programs" (Fortune et al., 2006, p. 235). Research placements focus on the knowledge and skills associated with research and provide opportunities to do 'hands-on' research (Council of Deans of Health, 2021).

The use of these models increased exponentially during the COVID-19 pandemic to ensure that students still had learning opportunities, when the number of placements plummeted but governments still expected students to graduate and join the workforce on time (Dario and Simic, 2021). However, these models of placement are not new and were documented in the literature more than a decade before the COVID-19 pandemic (e.g., Hall et al., 1996; Fortune et al., 2006; Lee, 2011). Early adopters of these models are clear that their value lies in the learning opportunities they offer students and not in filling the gaps resulting from a shortfall of placement provision (Fortune et al., 2006; Fortune and McKinstry, 2012; Beveridge and Pentland, 2020). For example, Ashley et al. (2022, p. 1) observed that "combining clinical and academic work through engagement with research can lead to benefits in terms of the quality, safety and efficacy of patient care". Competencies about evidence-based practice and research are embedded in the proficiency standards of professional and regulatory bodies, which means that project and research placements contribute as much to students' learning as other models of placement (Council of Deans of Health, 2021). As such, they are a valuable addition to the practice-based learning toolbox (Angus et al., 2022), especially as early engagement in research activities is also beneficial (Deal et al., 2016) (Figure 10.1).

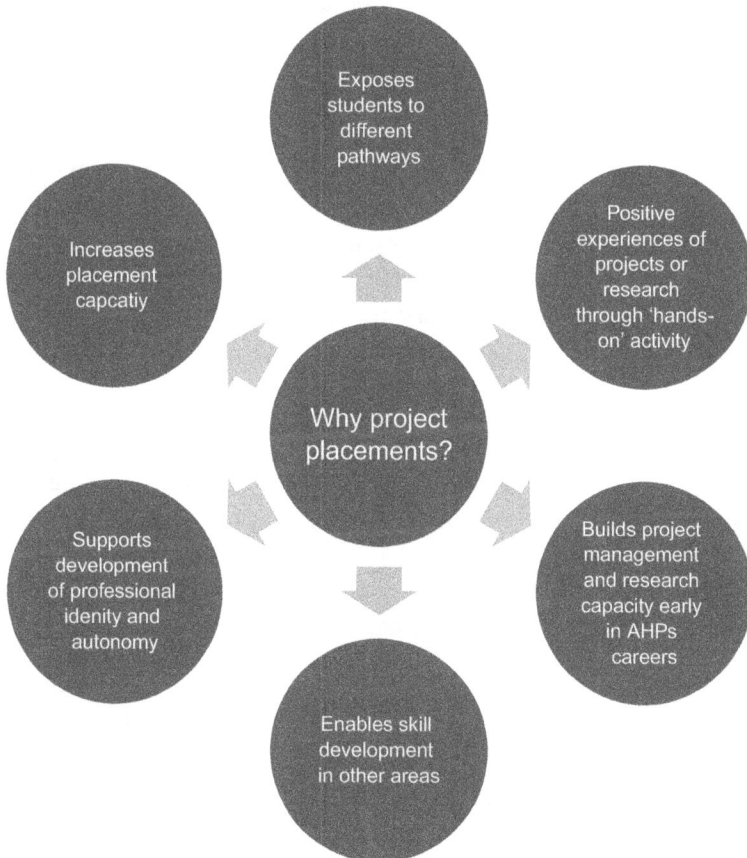

Figure 10.1 A summary of the benefits of project and research placements

A project placement is a model of placement whereby the student, either on their own or in peer-assisted learning groups (see Chapter 4), undertakes a practice-related project to develop skills in project management as the focus of their placement (Fortune et al., 2006; Beveridge and Pentland, 2020). They provide:

> *an opportunity for students to consider how their studies articulate theory with policy and practice; a consideration of ethical perspectives within their placement settings; developing a structured 'action plan' to work to and report back on; opportunities to apply theories of reflection on a regular basis in ways that inform their practice.*
>
> (Thompson, 2017, p. 414)

WHAT IS A RESEARCH PLACEMENT?

Concomitantly, in a research placement, the student – either on their own or in peer-assisted learning groups (see Chapter 4) – works on a practice-related research study as the focus of their placement. Research placements involve students developing and enhancing their research knowledge, skills and experience by working with a researcher to conduct a research study and can cover different types of research (Council of Deans of Health, 2021). A study by Angus et al. (2022, p. 4) gives the following indication of the range of ways students can be involved in these types of placements.

> *Some students worked on standalone projects, while others made contributions to larger projects, such as collecting data for a specific time period in a longer study. Fifteen projects had individual student allocations, and three projects had students working in groups of two, three or four. Student research involvement ranged from taking part solely in data collection, to active participation in numerous other project activities such as protocol development, ethics application, data analysis and dissemination of results.*

Dario and Simic (2021, p. 235) described "clinical research placements" as placements "whereby students are integrated in research projects that involve the delivery of evidence-based care . . . to build students' clinical skills and graduate qualities".

EVIDENCE BASE

To understand the evidence for project and research placements a rapid review was undertaken (Tricco et al., 2017) (Box 10.1). Of the 511 articles identified, 115 were duplicates, leaving 396 articles for title and abstract screening. Following screening for relevance, 17 articles were included. Of these, one focused on project placements in higher education generally (Thompson, 2017), one was multi-professional (Ashley et al., 2022), two focused on the allied health professions (Beveridge and Pentland, 2020; Angus et al., 2022), three were from specific allied health professions – occupational therapy (Fortune and McKinstry, 2012), physiotherapy (Dario and Simic, 2021) and speech and language therapy (Hopkins et al., 2022) – and one each came from geography (Tweed and Boast, 2011), medicine (Rocheteau, 2017) and pharmacy (Noble et al., 2022). Two were from social work (Hall et al., 1996; Calderwood and Rizzo, 2023a) and the remainder (n = 5) from nursing (Lee, 2011; Harrison, 2014; Naylor et al., 2014; Burrow, 2022; Lee et al., 2023). Citation searching identified three more relevant articles (Prigg and McKenzie, 2002; Fortune et al., 2006; James et al., 2016). Just over half of the literature is non-empirical (n = 11), confirming that the topic is under-researched (Beveridge and Pentland, 2020; Ashley et al., 2022) and demonstrating that project and research placement models are viable and a valuable learning experience (e.g., Dario and Simic, 2021; Lee et al., 2023).

BOX 10.1   SEARCH STRATEGY FOR THE RAPID REVIEW (CONDUCTED 24 NOVEMBER 2023)

AMED, British Education Index, CINAHL Complete, ERIC, Health Source: Nursing/Academic Edition and Medline were searched using the following search terms.

#1: Research placements	60,283
#2: Project placements	10,176
#3: #1 *or* #2	66,529
#4: Allied health professionals	38,941
#5: #4 *and* #3	472
#1: "Research placements"	27
#2: "Project placements"	12
#3: #1 *and* #2	39

DESIGN PRINCIPLES OF PROJECT AND RESEARCH PLACEMENTS

The literature has been analysed thematically and mapped to the author's experience of delivering project and research placements (see EmpowerAge™

practice example later in this chapter) to outline the design principles for these models of placement. These principles should be read in conjunction with Chapter 4 about peer-assisted learning because, whilst these models can be offered as learning experiences to individual students, our recommendation is that peer-assisted learning will provide students with an optimal learning experience because of the benefits of peer support (Lee et al., 2017; Ashley et al., 2022). It also enables the placement to run more smoothly from the practice educator's perspective.

Rationale for choice of model of placement

The first consideration is: why choose this model of placement? Calderwood and Rizzo (2023a, p. 140) are noticeably clear that these placements are "more than just a research assistant position focused on data analysis". Meanwhile, "As with other practice learning experiences, it should provide students with an opportunity to achieve their learning outcomes and to enhance their professional skills, understanding and employability" (Council of Deans of Health, 2021, p. 4). Placements are primarily a learning experience; the project or research study is the medium for learning, not the focus, and contributing to learning is often why practice educators are attracted to offering project and research placements (Dario and Simic, 2021; Angus et al., 2022). It must be explicit from the outset that conducting the project or research study can support the competencies and learning outcomes that the student must achieve (Fortune et al., 2006; Lee et al., 2023).

Approach to supervision

The importance of the student–practice educator relationship

Supervision is a key mechanism for student learning on placement (Dancza et al., 2023). In developing your approach, it may be helpful to think about how to enable learning and encourage greater student-directed learning (Prigg and McKenzie, 2002). (See Chapter 4 for ideas for supporting peer learning, and Chapter 5 for long-arm supervision). In relation to project and research placements, the literature offers the following useful insights.

Practice educator support is crucial (Beveridge and Pentland, 2020). "It is the [practice educator's] responsibility to provide a 'secure base' for the students' learning, and in such an environment the student becomes free to explore the professional world" (Calderwood and Rizzo, 2023a, p. 140). The success of such placements depends on supportive supervision from the practice educator (Fortune and McKinstry, 2012; Calderwood and Rizzo, 2023a), and this means availability of practice educators is important (Fortune and McKinstry, 2012). As one student observed, "The biggest thing that I think that I am taking away from this placement that means a lot to me is the mentorship that I received from [the practice educator]" (Calderwood and Rizzo, 2023a, p. 140).

Attributes and skills of a practice educator

As a practice educator, "you need to be able to motivate, develop and inspire others, take into account students' learning needs, and be approachable and encourage students to ask questions" (Naylor et al., 2014, p. 40). Students appreciate a practice educator being "genuine, passionate, approachable, open to communication, a role model, engaged, and caring" (Calderwood and Rizzo, 2023a, p. 140). To be a skilled practice educator, it is important to understand what is involved in being a practice educator and, if you do not have experience, attend practice educator training (Dario and Simic, 2021).

It is a balance

With project and research placements, practice educators spend less time directly supervising students because students work together on agreed tasks, but it does do require a careful balance between facilitating independence and supporting learning. This is because:

> There is a danger that practice educators might believe that offering a self-directed project placement means not having to spend time with students. However, self-direction is effective only when it is supported; therefore, the amount of time spent with students needs to be negotiated according to the individual needs of both practice educators and students.
>
> (Prigg and McKenzie, 2002, p. 233)

It is also possible to put too much emphasis on task completion rather than supporting the student to develop as a professional. Teaching students to be efficient and proficient researchers (or project managers) is often more important than completing the project (Goodlet and Nailor, 2020).

Manage your expectations as a practice educator

It is important for practice educators to maintain realistic expectations about students' skills and not make any assumptions about their baseline knowledge, even if they have prior project management or research experience (Goodlet and Nailor, 2020). As Angus et al. (2022, p. 5) found:

> *Several participants had anticipated that students would have higher capabilities than they exhibited. In particular, the extent of clinical skills needed for conducting the specified [project-related] tasks. For example, clinicians expected students to have more competency identifying patient eligibility, extracting patient data from clinical records and interpreting this for accuracy and study relevance according to inclusion criteria.*

Although professionals recognise the limited clinical ability of students who are still developing their professional practice skills, they do not always make the same allowances for project management and research skills (Angus et al., 2022). This means that a practice educator needs to evaluate each student's competency and the use this information to support them in develop learning plans to enable successful in engagement in the project or study.

Facilitating student learning

Students find it hard "dealing with unclear [practice educator] expectations, limited time with [practice educators] and [practice educators] not being aware of the evaluation procedure" (Prigg and McKenzie, 2002, p. 233). Therefore, it is important to not assume knowledge and check with students early on. Anticipate having to demonstrate skills at least once and having to check on the students work initially (Goodlet and Nailor, 2020). Lee's description illustrates the support needed:

> *I was given specific learning objectives tailored to the ward. I was unsure how I was going to achieve these objectives as I had not been in this type of environment before. My mentor helped me identify what I needed to do.*
> (Lee, 2011, p. 29)

Practice educators need to be explicit about the learning that is taking place, and to make links between the professional skills being acquired and their application to practice (Prigg and McKenzie, 2002). It also helps to manage expectations, e.g., outline roles; explain if there is limited opportunity for client contact; decide who is doing what, if working collaboratively; and agree standards the students are working to. However, some of this will evolve over the project (Angus et al., 2022).

Mode of delivery

These placements can be delivered face to face or as a technology-enabled placement in an online, virtual or hybrid format (see Chapter 6). The decision about which to choose will be dictated by the nature of the project; for example, a literature review is likely to be easier to conduct online, but enabling students learning (as previously described) will also inform the decision about the mode of delivery.

Planning and preparation

Project and research placements are not time neutral (Fortune and McKinstry, 2012). Organisation is key because they require planning and preparation (Hall et al., 1996; Ashley et al., 2022). The investment pays off for student and practice educator alike because it helps to reduce anxiety which can be heighted if a student is not familiar with project management or research process (Noble et al., 2022). Planning requires the following.

IDENTIFYING A PROJECT OR STUDY

The first step is to identify an appropriate project (Goodlet and Nailor, 2020). It is not like a dissertation; the project or study is generated by the practice educator rather than by the student (Angus et al., 2022). It may be helpful to think about projects you would have liked to have progressed but have not had time to do so, or service needs that cannot be prioritised without additional support. Considering the following points helps with the decision about what is viable.

- **Timeline**: Placements vary in terms of length, so it needs to be do-able in the time.
- **Placement setting**: Where will the project be located?
- **Number of students**: Will it involve one or multiple students?
- **Stakeholders buy-in**: Is there local support for the project?
- **Ethical constraints**: A research project needs to comply with ethical requirements. Is approval needed for any potential changes to research activities?
- **Learning experience**: Will it provide an authentic learning experience? (Dario and Simic, 2021). Will it provide a relevant learning experience for the student level? (Prigg and McKenzie, 2002). Will the student(s) have some degree of client/consumer contact?

It may be that the student is not able to complete entire process and that sequential placements are needed to complete a project or study.

MAP ONTO LEARNING OUTCOMES

Once the project has been decided upon, the next step is to focus on learning outcomes, so it is explicit how the project or research study will enable the student(s) to achieve them (Fortune and McKinstry, 2012; Thompson, 2017). Equally, students need to have clearly defined tasks and outputs, and that these are associated with specific deadlines and that the work corresponds to the learning outcomes and hours associated with the module, although this may require some creativity with interpreting how learning outcome are applied to this non-clinical setting.

PLAN PLACEMENT EXPERIENCE

When the project or study has been devised, you can start to plan the placement activities, especially if it is a short placement, to maximise the students' learning experience (Thompson, 2017). It is important to be realistic about what is achievable in the time (Angus et al., 2022). The plan should include opportunities to acclimatise, e.g., understand organisational culture (Fortune and McKinstry, 2012), and socialise professionally, as well as conduct the project (Beveridge and Pentland, 2020), and it is helpful to remember that the project or study will make more sense to the student as time progresses (Fortune and McKinstry, 2012). Students have observed the following.

- Initially, they were overwhelmed with the perceived responsibility (Hopkins et al., 2022).
- Having a basic understanding of the concepts before starting can might make the first weeks less daunting (Burrow, 2022).
- The benefit of step-by-step learning (Fortune and McKinstry, 2012).
- A structured approach is important, especially at the beginning so that students "feel safe" and gain confidence. Being disorganised does not help (Thompson, 2017).

Forward planning, particularly having dates in the diary for meetings from the start, helps students to feel secure. It may be helpful to provide placement related information before the placement for students to familiarise themselves with (Prigg and McKenzie, 2002; Naylor et al., 2014). The sort of learning resources to consider preparing include a placement manual, orientation session, supervision arrangements and training opportunities, such as GCP training (Burrow, 2022) or the online Physiotherapy Evidence Database (PEDro) Scale training programme (Dario and Simic, 2021), tailored to the project or study and the tasks the students will be involved in. Anticipating potential challenges – for example, how variability in recruitment rate can affect students' activities and how this might be resolved (Dario and Simic, 2021) – is another part of planning the placement experience.

Implementing placement

This essentially involves putting enacting your plans and preparations, namely the following.

- **Creating sense of belonging**: The feeling of being part of a team and getting involved with colleagues is appreciated by students because it supports the development of their confidence and independence (Thompson, 2017; Hopkins et al., 2022). This means that they need support with relationship building. Chapter 3 on equality, diversity, inclusion and belonging has guidance on facilitating an inclusive placement experience. Students are active partners in the process of project and research placements. Personal development planning is an essential element in achieving this, and reflection can support this activity (Dancza et al., 2023).
- **Creating a learning environment**: Students and educators work together as a team on these placements. This means that there is a need for practice educators to set and/or negotiate core tasks for student to work on (Council of Deans of Health, 2021), which requires careful time management. The educator also applies their approach to supervision (as previously discusseed); supervision sessions may be offered individually, in groups or a mix of both. Students learning is fostered through the following.
- **Induction (or orientation) session**: Students will need an induction or orientation session, before starting their project or study, to achieve the following.

  - Set shared ground rules for communication and 'checking in', including what to do if the student experiences challenges on the placement.
  - Clarify roles, goals, timelines, expectations and mechanisms for feedback (both formative and summative assessment).
  - Provide an overview of the project (including any ethical issues if relevant).
  - Outline any education sessions, e.g., tutorials.

- Describe the planned scope of the student's involvement.
- Help students to understand they are "serving two agendas"; doing the project or research work as well as meeting the placement learning outcomes (Tweed and Boast, 2011, p. 612).
- Describe the criteria for success, including what the outcome is for the project or study, so students know what they are working towards.
- Discuss how the project or study will help the student(s) to meet the learning outcomes.

- **Student support**: As the placement progresses and the practice educator has a greater sense of the students and their learning needs, they may need to adapt their approach to support the student's learning (see Chapter 3). All the usual support mechanisms are in place for students on project and research placements as others. Students should be strongly encouraged to use these if needed.
- **Monitoring progress**: In line with assessment and feedback principles, once the placement is underway it is important to carefully monitor the project or study's progress and evaluate whether the learning outcomes are being achieved. If adaptations are needed that should be implemented as soon as possible in discussion with the students so that they fully understand the implications.
- **Dissemination**: For motivated students, practice educators should encourage formal sharing of the project outcome or research findings (Goodlet and Nailor, 2020). As part of EmpowerAge™ (see practice example 2 later in this chapter) dissemination, I presented with students at the World Federation of Occupational Therapists Congress (Bannigan et al., 2022). Students should be advised of any potential opportunities for authorship, but it should be recognised that data collection alone is not sufficient to merit authorship (Goodlet and Nailor, 2020).

Post-placement

The focus of this phase is debriefing and evaluation to develop and grow the placement experience. It involves using feedback from students, service users and carers (if applicable), and staff to improve future placements. Feedback should be collected anonymously to allow students to comment openly as opposed to having to give direct feedback to their educator (Naylor et al., 2014). Any changes needed can be implemented with the next group of students to undertake the placement. For example, Harrison (2014) described how they reviewed their placement feedback form and developed a revised version. The placement experience may highlight additional learning needs, in which case the practice educator can signpost to learning resources for the students to engage in post-placement to nurture and develop their learning. Students have highlighted that they need to believe that their projects are valued by the workplace; otherwise, they were less likely to be motivated to complete the project (Prigg and McKenzie, 2002). This means practice educators need to communicate to their students the value of their contribution and how the project or study is recognised by the workplace (Prigg and McKenzie, 2002). It is important to plan for sustainability so that a programme of work is developed that enables project and research programmes to be offered over time rather than a one-off placement. This increases impact and is a better return on investment. The quality of the placement is important, which is why all placements including project and research placements are audited, at least annually, as part of the higher education institution's quality assurance processes to ensure that they are safe and facilitate quality learning experiences.

PRACTICE EXAMPLES

Practice educators often want evidence that a model they have not used before 'works' before trying it (OTalk, 2022). It is reassuring to learn that practice educators concerns and issues lessen once they engage in new forms of practice education (Beveridge and Pentland, 2020). To support this, examples of success stories of project and research placements have been included to inspire use of these models, if they have not been already. There were six examples included in the Council of Deans of Health (2021) report about research placements, and Dario and Simic (2021) provided a table of examples of learning and teaching opportunities for students and clinicians/researchers involved in their clinical research placement pilot. We have deliberately provided the following examples to increase the number and range of examples available.

- **Example 1 – Major trauma project placement in paramedicine**: This project placement could be described as 'innovation born out of necessity'. One of the placements that paramedicine students at Glasgow Caledonian University need to undertake is a cross-sector placement to observe the patient journey beyond the front door. However, due the pressures on services because of COVID-19, it was difficult for them to offer a two-week placement. To overcome these challenges, a split placement – involving a clinical week and a project week – was developed. During the clinical week, students spend time with the major trauma team; in their project week, students undertake a project based on something they regarded as key learning that would be useful for other learners. The project output can be a case study, a leaflet, a poster or an infographic and is shared with their peers to broaden their learning. These placements are not without their challenges, such as the coordination of providing staff across the clinical and academic settings to manage the two parts of the placement and helping students understand the level of work commensurate with a week's project. With that said, the placement has been invaluable in developing students' skills in reflection, increasing 'peer-to-peer' learning and broadening the exposure of students to major trauma setting without increasing demands on the services.

- **Example 2 – EmpowerAge™ (public health)**: EmpowerAge™ is an occupation-based manualised intervention developed to promote healthy ageing. It has become a programme of work – to develop and evaluate a complex intervention – that has involved several project and research placements to date. Students have conducted a review, developed a draft manual and developed a strategy for public engagement and patient and public involvement work. Future placements planned include acceptability testing, feasibility testing and testing effectiveness. The placements are offered as hybrid placements, involving one practice educator and up to six students (but always an even number of students to enable students to work in pairs as peer learners). Students and educators meet daily (which saves time in the long run), and a mix of group and individual supervision is used. Students start the placement with a reading day focused on key texts, followed by an education day facilitated by the placement educator to orientate them to the project or study and the students negotiate the work and develop a time plane with support.
- **Example 3 – The effectiveness of the Early Years version of the 'Word Aware' programme in supporting the development of vocabulary knowledge** (Hopkins et al., 2022): Two student speech and language therapists, who were completing their final-year placement, participated as researchers in this mixed-methods study. Following training, the students were involved in the following.

  - Delivering the 'Word Aware' intervention.
  - Blind pre-test assessments.
  - An additional two-hour briefing session at the university to outline the procedure of data collection and management, and included instructions for accurate test administration.
  - Meeting with the teaching staff every week to review, discuss progress and identify any challenges that could be resolved.
  - Supporting the delivery of 'Word Aware'.
  - An afternoon debriefing session midway through the intervention with the students to review progress and to offer solutions to any challenges faced.

- **Example 4 – Development and pilot implementation of a training framework to prepare and integrate pharmacy students into a multicentre hospital research study** (Noble et al., 2022): Pharmacy students collected data from 38 patients and were involved in patient screening processes, interviewing, data collection and analysis. The placement enabled students to obtain skills in (1) literature searching; (2) maintaining patient confidentiality; (3) interviewing patients; (4) obtaining data from medical records; (5) communicating with patients and clinicians; and (6) the use of clinical information to predict medication related harm risk. A framework was developed to guide the separation of roles and responsibilities between students and researchers. See Noble et al. (2022) for full details of the framework.

SUMMING UP

In essence, project and research placements have a pedigree that pre-dates COVID-19, but they have not been widely adopted. The current climate in health and social care, described in Chapter 2, have supported their wider use. This overview of the literature, key principles and practice examples provides a starting point for those new to these models. If you are still unsure how to get started, particularly with identifying a project or study, do not be afraid to ask for help. For example, in the UK, the Royal College of Occupational Therapists hosts a placement café and RCOT Research Connect, but if you do not have access to a resource such as this, another strategy is to liaise with your local higher education institution.

FUTURE DIRECTIONS

The future of these placements depends on increasing their availability and uptake. This may be achieved by getting students to talk about their experience to encourage others to offer or take up research placements (Council of Deans of Health, 2021). The focus of project and research placements has tended to be on discrete placements to date. The value of these placements may increase if they can be deployed to facilitate programmes of work overtime. As well as promoting the sustainability of this model of placement, it may provide a better return on investment for the effort involved in setting up the initial placement, as well as a richer learning experience. Research is needed to test the veracity of this conjecture and to get a better understanding of these placements across the allied health professions. If programmes of work can be achieved through this model of placement, they may become a means to progress project and research work more quickly (Angus et al., 2022).

A FINAL WORD

Although these models of placement pre-date the COVID-19 pandemic, I had never participated in one before then. To date, my work on EmpowerAge™ (see practice example 2 in this chapter) has spanned four placements and involved working with 32 students. I have been inspired by – and learnt from – the students I have worked with. This experience has enhanced my working life and enabled me to develop a new programme of work that I might not otherwise have been able to. Others who have engaged in these types of placements have had similarly rewarding and fulfilling experiences (e.g., Lee, 2011; Tweed and Boast, 2011; Dario and Simic, 2021; Angus et al., 2022). Hopefully, whether you are a student or educator, you feel inspired to consider trying these models of practice-based learning, if you have not already.

RESOURCES

- Project placements resource for allied health professional practice educators developed by Caty O'Connell, available at https://learn.nes.nhs.scot/62593
- Project placements resource from the University of Queensland, available at https://otpecq.group.uq.edu.au/education-placements/placement-options-and-models/project-placements
- Detailed tips for conducting clinical research with students (Goodlet and Nailor, 2020).
- A six-stage process they used for implementing project placements (Prigg and McKenzie, 2002).
- A description of developing a research placement (Calderwood and Rizzo, 2023b).

REFERENCES

Angus, R. L., Hattingh, H. L. and Weir, K. A. (2022). Experiences of hospital allied health professionals in collaborative student research projects: A qualitative study. *BMC Health Services Research*, *22*, p. 729. https://doi.org/10.1186/s12913-022-08119-7

Ashley, A., Sutton, E., MacKinnon, H. and Lotto, R. (2022). Challenges and opportunities in delivering multi-institutional and multi-professional research placements. *British Journal of Cardiac Nursing*, *17*(5), pp. 1–4. https://doi.org/10.12968/bjca.2022.0028

Bannigan, K., Alderson, S., Bird, A., Hyland, M. G., Lovett, C., McMenemy, L. A. and Smith, S. (2022). Occupational therapy and the transition from work to retirement: A rapid review. *Proceedings of the 18th World Federation of Occupational Therapists Congress*, Paris, 28–31 August. Available at: https://archive.wfot.org/wfot2022/programme/full-programme.html

Beveridge, J. and Pentland, D. (2020). A mapping review of models of practice education in allied health and social care professions. *British Journal of Occupational Therapy*, *83*(8), pp. 488–513. https://doi.org/10.1177/030802262090432

Burrow, H. (2022). Applying ethics in a real-world setting on a research placement. *Nursing Standard*, *37*(12), pp. 27–28. https://doi.org/10.7748/ns.37.12.27.s15

Calderwood, K. A. and Rizzo, L. N. (2023a). Co-creating a transformative learning environment through the student-supervisor relationship: Results of a social work field placement duo-ethnography. *Journal of Transformative Education*, *21*(1), pp. 138–156. https://doi.org/10.1177/15413446221079590

Calderwood, K. A. and Rizzo, L. N. (2023b). Meeting learning objectives in an in-house research placement: Results of a student-supervisor duo-ethnography. *Social Work Education*, *42*(8), pp. 1327–1343. https://doi.org/10.1080/02615479.2021.2021173

Council of Deans of Health. (2021). *Becoming research confident: Research placements in pre-registration nursing, midwifery, and health programmes in the UK*. Available at: https://www.councilofdeans.org.uk/wp-content/uploads/2021/07/010621-research-placement-report-FINAL-updated-220621.pdf (Accessed 24 November 2023).

Dancza, K., Volkert, A. and Tempest, S. (2023). *Supervision for Occupational Therapy: Practical Guidance for Supervisors and Supervisees*. Abingdon, Oxon: Routledge.

Dario, A. and Simic, M. (2021). Innovative physiotherapy clinical education in response to the COVID-19 pandemic with a clinical research placement model. *Journal of Physiotherapy*, *67*(4), pp. 235–237. https://doi.org/10.1016/j.jphys.2021.08.008.

Deal, E. N., Stranges, P. M., Maxwell, W. D., Bacci, J., Ashjian, E. J., DeRemer, D. L., Kane-Gill, S. L., Norgard, N. B., Dombrowski, L., Parker, R. B. and American College of Clinical Pharmacy. (2016). The importance of research and scholarly activity in pharmacy training. *Pharmacotherapy*, *36*, pp. e200–e205. https://doi.org/10.1002/phar.1864

Fortune, T., Farnworth, L. and McKinstry, C. (2006). Project focussed fieldwork: Core business of fieldwork fillers? *Australian Occupational Therapy Journal*, *53*, pp. 233–236. https://doi.org/10.1111/j.1440-1630.2006.00562.x

Fortune, T. and McKinstry, C. (2012). Project-based fieldwork: Perspectives of graduate entry students and project sponsors. *Australian Occupational Therapy Journal*, *59*(4), pp. 265–275. https://doi.org/10.1111/j.1440-1630.2012.01026.x

Goodlet, K. J. and Nailor, M. D. (2020). Involving pharmacy students in clinical research: Tips and best practices. *American Journal of Health-System Pharmacy*, *77*(23), pp. 1946–1948. https://doi.org/10.1093/ajhp/zxaa290

Hall, J. A., Jensen, G. V., Fortney, M. A., Sutter, J., Locher, J. and Cayner, J. J. (1996). Education of staff and students in health care settings: Integrating practice and research. *Social Work in Health Care*, *24*(1/2), pp. 93–113. https://doi.org/10.1300/J010v24n01_06

Harrison, M. (2014). Enhancing student nurses' experience through cardiac research placements. *British Journal of Cardiac Nursing*, *9*(9), pp. 453–456. https://doi.org/10.12968/bjca.2014.9.9.453

Hedley, C. (2023). *Traditional vs non-traditional practice education . . . what's in a word?* Available at: https://www.rcot.co.uk/traditional-vs-non-traditional-practice-education%E2%80%A6what%E2%80%99s-word?hash=n21Wwees9a7lGUmlGmLap_trN_cORGFNtKCdBOdSI0Q&utm_campaign=1290682_Scottish%20Western%20Region%20general%20April%202023&utm_medium=email&utm_source=dotdigital&dm_i=6Q9X,RNWA,3IU6HX,3GC6W,1 (Accessed 24 November 2023).

Hopkins, T., Harrison, E., Coyne-Umfreville, E. and Packer, M. (2022). A pilot study exploring the effectiveness of a whole-school intervention targeting receptive vocabulary in the early years: Findings from a mixed method study involving students as part of a practice-based research placement. *Child Language Teaching and Therapy*, *38*(2), pp. 212–229. https://doi.org/10.1177/02656590221088210

James, B., Beattie, M., Shepherd, A., Armstrong, L. and Wilkinson, J. (2016). Time, fear and transformation: Student nurses' experiences of doing a practicum (quality improvement project) in practice. *Nurse Education in Practice*, *19*, pp. 70–78. https://doi.org/10.1016/j.nepr.2016.05.004

Lee, B. J. (2011). Starting out research placement offered a unique learning opportunity. *Nursing Standard*, *25*(22), p. 29.

Lee, B. J., Rhodes, N. J., Scheetz, M. H. and McLaughlin, M. M. (2017). Engaging pharmacy students in research through near-peer training. *American Journal of Pharmaceutical Education*, *81*(9), p. 6340. https://doi.org/10.5688/ajpe6340

Lee, G. A., Raleigh, M. and Robbins, K. (2023). Research placements: Are they a suitable alternative for student nurses? *British Journal of Nursing*, *32*(3), pp. 126–128. https://doi.org/10.12968/bjon.2023.32.3.126

Naylor, G. A., Hanson, A., Evely, J., Little, M. and VanEker, D. (2014). Nursing student placements in clinical research. *Nursing Standard*, *29*(2), pp. 37–43. https://doi.org/10.7748/ns.29.2.37.e8683

Noble, A., Raleigh, R., Page, A. and Hattingh, H. L. (2022). Development and pilot implementation of a training framework to prepare and integrate pharmacy students into a multicentre hospital research study. *Pharmacy*, *10*(3), p. 57. https://doi.org/10.3390/pharmacy10030057

OTalk. (2022). *#OTalk – Tuesday 25th October 2022 – everyone needs a PAL hosted by @AnitavAHP @KatrinaBannigan*. Available at: https://otalk.co.uk/2022/10/19/otalk-25th-october-2022-everyone-needs-a-pal-hosted-by-anitavahp-katrinabannigan/ (Accessed 26 November 2023).

Prigg, A. and McKenzie, L. (2002). Project placements for undergraduate occupational therapy students, design, implementation and evaluation. *Occupational Therapy International*, *9*(3), pp. 210–236. https://doi.org/10.1002/oti.166

Rocheteau, E. (2017). How to organise a summer research placement. *The British Medical Journal*, 385. https://doi.org/10.1136/sbmj.j2888

Thompson, D. W. (2017). How valuable is "short project" placement experience to higher education students? *Journal of Further and Higher Education*, *41*(3), pp. 413–424. https://doi.org/10.1080/0309877X.2015.1117601

Tricco, A. C., Langlois, E. V. and Straus, S. E. (2017). *Rapid reviews to strengthen health policy and systems: A practical guide*. World Health Organization. Available at: https://ahpsr.who.int/publications/i/item/2017-08-10-rapid-reviews-to-strengthen-health-policy-and-systems-a-practical-guide (Accessed 25 November 2023).

Tweed, F. and Boast, R. (2011). Reviewing the "research placement" as a means of enhancing student learning and stimulating research activity. *Journal of Geography in Higher Education*, *35*(4), pp. 599–615. https://doi.org/10.1080/03098265.2011.559579

Chapter 11

Student-led clinics

Sandra Robertson, Emma Green and Katrina Bannigan

CHAPTER OVERVIEW

Student-led clinics are a model of practice-based learning that involve students taking responsibility for the organisation and delivery of a clinic. This chapter provides an overview of student-led clinics, outlining the key design features as well as exploring the rationale for establishing a student-led clinic. The chapter also highlights the opportunities student-led clinics provide, such as interprofessional education and collaboration, along with development of professional and clinical skills, as well as the potential challenges, such as funding and operational costs. Real-life examples of student-led clinics and an overview of future directions for this model of practice-based learning are presented.

CHAPTER OBJECTIVES

The objectives of this chapter are the following.

- A definition and rationale for student-led clinics to support allied health practice–based learning.
- An overview of the evidence base for student-led clinics, outlining the benefits and challenges of developing and implementing a student-led clinic.
- Considerations of the design principles of setting up, implementing and sustaining a student-led clinic.
- Real-world case examples of student-led clinics.

DOI: 10.4324/9781003411765-11

INTRODUCTION

Student-led clinics are a model of practice-based learning whereby students "take primary responsibility for organising and leading a health care service" (Wynne and Cooper, 2021, p. 2958). Student-led clinics aim to create real-world learning experiences reflective of health and social care practice, whereby students are supported by clinical educators and which are of value to service users (Kavanagh et al., 2015; Hopkins et al., 2022). Provision of quality and sustainable practice-based learning opportunities are essential to develop the future workforce (Chartered Society of Physiotherapy, 2023). Student-led clinics enable students to develop an understanding of their own role and scope of practice, and the role and scope of other professionals, as well as how to work as part of an interprofessional team (Hopkins et al., 2022). Schutte et al. (2018, p. 122) highlight that student-led clinics have emerged as "innovative educational platforms that promote interprofessional education while also addressing the healthcare needs of underserved communities". Student-led clinics are offered to populations that would not routinely be able to access healthcare services (Sick et al., 2017). Since the 1960s in the United States, student-led clinics have been well established for medical students with the main purpose of providing "free primary health care services to those who are poor and uninsured" (Maple et al., 2023). There is also evidence of the establishment of student-led clinics in Europe, Asia, Africa and Australia (Maple et al., 2023). Student-led clinics provide creative opportunities for collaborative education, community-engaged learning, social responsibility, and early practical clinical training and can deliver services to marginalised populations including the homeless (Schutte et al., 2015; Simpson and Long, 2007).

MODEL OF PLACEMENT

Student-led clinics provide an inventive way of meeting the demand for practice-based learning opportunities (Wynne and Cooper, 2019), as they enable students to run clinics within a university context while being supported by academics and/or practice educators (Beveridge and Pentland, 2020). They "provide appropriate care to a population of need whilst providing work-integrated learning for students" (Walpola and Schneider, 2018, p. 473) and an environment in which students can communicate, collaborate and share the responsibilities associated with the delivery of patient care (Yap et al., 2024). They are structured to meet the needs of learners, as well as address unmet community health needs (Kent et al., 2016). They also provide an environment that supports and develops key areas of health professional practice, such as clinical reasoning and implementing treatment and management (Abrey et al., 2022). They are also a valuable opportunity for health and social care professional students to undertake clinical education placements in environments other than traditional hospital settings while also providing an opportunity for interprofessional learning experiences (Haines et al., 2014) whereby students can "learn with, from, and about each other through interprofessional practice in a real-world setting" (Hopkins et al., 2022, p. 235).

There are several definitions of student-led clinics, although not one that is universally accepted (Maple et al., 2023). Briggs and Fronek (2020, p. 238) describe student-led clinics as health clinics where "students deliver services under the supervision of qualified educators who are appropriately licensed or accredited". Simpson and Long (2007) broaden the definition to a "mode of health care delivery in which medical, nursing and/or health care professional students take primary responsibility for the logistics and operational management of the clinic". The focus of student-led clinics is the student as lead provider of patient care while being supervised by a qualified clinical educator as students take on the responsibility for areas such as logistical operations and administration (Abrey et al., 2022; Gillies et al., 2019). Whilst student-led clinics are typically located as part of a community campus, but they can also be found as part of an outreach clinic or community health clinic where students are able to develop their confidence in engaging with diverse populations (Abrey et al., 2022; Geelhoed et al., 2019).

EVIDENCE BASE FOR STUDENT-LED CLINICS

The evidence base for student-led clinics within allied health is in its infancy. This model of placement is not widely utilised in practice, but there are some examples in the literature, from a Western Global North context, e.g., the United States and Australia. These examples tend to be interprofessional in nature – i.e., Haines et al. (2014), Gustafsson et al. (2016), Kent et al. (2016), Hu et al. (2018), Sick et al. (2017), Hopkins et al. (2022), Maple et al. (2023) – with a few examples being uni-professional, namely osteopathy (Abrey et al., 2022) and physiotherapy (George et al., 2017; Sick et al., 2017; Geelhoed et al., 2019; Gillies et al., 2019). The types of student-led clinics evident within the evidence base were largely community health clinics (n = 7), including a musculoskeletal osteopathy clinic (Abrey et al., 2022), and interprofessional clinics (Haines et al., 2014; Gustafsson et al., 2016; George et al., 2017; Sick et al., 2017; Hopkins et al., 2022). The others were campus based (Kent et al., 2016; Hu et al., 2018), a clinic run as a component of an established network of student-run free healthcare clinics with multiple different professional services (Gillies et al., 2019) and a physiotherapy pro bono clinic in a homelessness shelter (Geelhoed et al., 2019). The research to date has focused on the learner's perceptions (Hu et al. (2018), attitudes (Sick et al., 2017) and experiences (Gustafsson et al., 2016). Abrey et al. (2022), and Geelhoed et al. (2019) researched the experiences and attitudes of both learners and practice educators towards student-led clinics. Other research noted from the literature included an economic evaluation (Haines et al., 2014), an evaluation of the value of the student-led clinic (Kent et al., 2016) and a study focused on the implementation of a student-led clinic (George et al., 2017).

Two reviews have been undertaken into student-led clinics, a rapid review by Hopkins et al. (2022) and a scoping review by Maple et al. (2023). Hopkins et al. (2022) aimed to explore the benefits to allied health students of participating in an interprofessional student-led clinic. It explored the benefits particularly for meeting interprofessional educational requirements, finding that student-led clinics do provide a valuable means of learners achieving outcomes related to interprofessional education, in terms of role and scope of professional roles, teamwork and patient-centred care. Maple et al.'s (2023) scoping review was focused on understanding whether school-based student-led clinics meet the required accreditation standards within Australia; using broad categories to define practice-based learning experiences, they concluded that school-based student-led clinics can provide valuable learning experiences for healthcare disciplines. However, the lack of guidance available led Maple et al. (2023) to suggest that higher education institutions trying to develop this model of practice-based learning should learn from the experiences of others. Due to the limited literature available, both these reviews were small in scale, and the potential value of student-led clinics for learners, practice educators and service users who access these services requires further research. With that said, some conclusions can be drawn as to the benefits and challenges of student-led clinics.

Benefits of student-led clinics

To date, most of the literature has evaluated the experiences and perception of learners within this type of placement setting. Student-led clinics are an attractive option for practice-based learning provision because of the benefits for students and practice educators. Students benefit from being able to work in real-life settings (Passmore et al., 2016; Yap et al., 2024) where they can assume responsibility for patients in areas such as preparing for consultations and being able to collaborate with other students and their clinical supervisors (Schutte et al., 2018). Students can develop interprofessional competencies including being able to develop communication skills to engage effectively with other professionals (Gillies et al., 2019). Gustafsson et al. (2016, p. 260) reported that participation in a student-led clinic enabled students to "validate their own role within the team while considering other professional's perspectives and approaches to achieving combined therapy goals". They also provide the opportunity for students to develop their confidence in areas such as being able to ask questions, gain assurance in relation to what their role and scope is within a team and that of other professionals, whilst also considering the importance of co-operation as part of interprofessional practice (Gustafsson et al., 2016; Hopkins et al., 2022). Student-led clinics enable students to learn how to work as part of an interprofessional team (Hopkins et al., 2022), which is important because collaborative practice is key to "safe, high quality, accessible, equitable, person/client-centred care and enhanced population health outcomes" (Interprofessional Education Collaborative, 2023, p. 15).

Passmore et al. (2016, p. 393) suggest being "exposed to marginalized patient populations, learning through interprofessional interactions, and being introduced to different patient care approaches" are also benefits of student engagement in a student-led clinic. The opportunity to work in a real-world healthcare setting supports students to develop their communication skills, strengthen their profession-specific skills and improve their confidence to work as part of an interprofessional team (Hopkins et al., 2022). George et al. (2017) also highlight the value of students participating in interprofessional education and collaborative practice while outlining that student-led clinics provide an opportunity for experimental learning and the development of leadership skills. A student-led clinic is an environment in which students can both display and naturally develop their leadership skills (Abrey et al., 2022). Responsibility for patients and other students, and authenticity in relation to the experience and collaboration with students, supervisors and student coordinators, all interact in a student-led clinic to enhance learning (Schutte et al., 2018). The experience of engaging in a student-led clinic is "extremely positive and meaningful" for students (Hu et al., 2018, p. 77).

From the perspective of educators, student-led clinics present a range of benefits including cultural competence, improved academic outcomes and students being in an environment in which they can develop aspects of their professional and ethical behaviours, consolidating their treatment skills and being able to work with individuals who they would be unlikely to gain experience with in more traditional placement settings (Abrey et al., 2022; Geelhoed et al., 2019; Maple et al., 2023). Other benefits for educators include establishing collaborations with partners in healthcare and the opportunity to provide placements for students (Tokolahi et al., 2021). As student-led clinics present an important opportunity to help "bridge gaps in both the health care and professional education systems" (George et al., 2017, p. 63), it allows providers to provide services to underserved populations by increasing student exposure to patients who may not normally be able to access healthcare services and the provision of authentic learning experiences (Geelhoed et al., 2019; George et al., 2017).

There are few studies evaluating the benefits of the student-led clinics from the perspective of service users accessing the services of student-led clinics, and this is a gap in the literature. Kent et al. (2016) is one notable exception; they evaluated the patient experience of their interprofessional clinic focused on delivering a service for community-dwelling older people who had recently been discharged from hospital and attended the clinic. Using a Patient Experience Questionnaire, they found that 64% (61 out of 96) were favourable in their perceived value of the student-led clinic.

Challenges associated with student-led clinics

While there are many benefits to student-led clinics in terms of the opportunities they present for students to develop skills in areas such as leadership, communication, teamwork and working with diverse communities, challenges have also been identified in the literature. Challenges relating to student-led clinics includes the perception of some students that clinics do not provide them with the opportunity to gain a wide range of experience in terms of the "problems and treatments regarded as important to their professional development" (Abrey et al., 2022, p. 2). They reported insufficient opportunity to develop their professional communication, the wide variety of problems experienced by patients, the number of patients, lack of cultural diversity and consultations not being authentic. In relation to consultations not being authentic, this presents a particular challenge because students may be treating a population that is healthy, which potentially does not prepare them to be able to work with patients who have more complex care needs (Abrey et al., 2022). In terms of working with other professionals, the student-led clinic environment can be challenging due to time pressures, the motivation of the clinical educators and the limited diversity of the patient population (George et al., 2017; Abrey et al., 2022). Equally, it is important that there are strategies put in place to enable professionals to work together because otherwise, interprofessional work may not take place (Hopkins et al., 2022). Other challenges in relation to student-led clinics focus on being able to balance the needs and goals of different stakeholders – namely the students, the patients and the university – whilst ensuring that the required risk assessment procedures are in place (George et al., 2017). Financial sustainability and the operational costs are also a challenge; student-led clinics present higher daily costs than more traditional models of practice-based learning such as hospital-based placements (Haines et al., 2014; Kent et al., 2016; Maple et al., 2023). Other issues highlighted were the space available within clinics, limited capacity for supervision, the time management of students, the number of students, available students being able to work effectively within a multidisciplinary team and the planning and management of student-led clinics (Maple et al., 2023).

DESIGN PRINCIPLES OF MODEL OF PLACEMENT

Student-led clinics involve several stakeholders and require careful planning and design to ensure they benefit students, meet needs of service users for whom they are developed and provide a sustainable model that can be resourced and maintained. Robust planning is required to address challenges associated with student-led clinics such as infrastructure, funding, the required level of supervisor time, management of student-related issues and facilitating interprofessional work (Maple et al., 2023). See Table 11.1 for a summary of design principles for student-led clinics.

Rationale for student-led clinic

There is a wide variety of reasons why education providers may wish to establish a student-led clinic as a model of practice-based learning. One is to address capacity issues and the shortage of suitable practice-based learning experiences in the real world; student-led clinics can provide an alternative safe and supportive learning environment (Abrey et al., 2022; Maple et al., 2023; Haines et al., 2014). There is also a need to increase the diversity of practice-based learning opportunities for students, and student-led clinics have the potential to address this, as well as enhancing the quality of education experienced by students (Abrey et al., 2022). Student-led clinics can provide a different approach to traditional practice-based learning settings (Maple et al., 2023), including uni-professional and interprofessional experiences.

Student-led clinics afford a range of learning opportunities that can be adapted to the stage and learning requirements of individuals or groups of students directed by expected learning outcomes. As student-led clinics offer a service for groups and communities, the setting reflects real-world practice for allied health and learning opportunities that can include the following.

- **Enhancing clinical skills and practical experience**: Student-led clinics offer students hands-on experience, which is a critical component of professional education. By directly engaging with patients, students improve their

Table 11.1 Design principles for student-led clinics

Rationale for choice of model of placement	• Student-led clinics provide an alternative to limited real-world practice opportunities, offering diverse, safe learning environments for students while addressing community health needs. • These clinics allow students to develop clinical skills, promote interprofessional teamwork and refine professionalism and ethical practices, preparing them for future healthcare roles. • Student-led clinics support reflective practice, self-assessment and continuous improvement, while also benefiting local communities by filling service gaps and supporting institutional missions.
Can the placement be supported as PAL?	• Typically, student-led clinics would be delivered with peer learning as a central educational approach. • Peer learning in student-led clinics encourages teamwork, mutual support and the development of effective communication skills essential for interprofessional practice. • Working alongside peers helps students build confidence, reflect on their practice and engage in problem solving through shared experiences and feedback. • Peer learning mirrors real-world healthcare settings, preparing students for collaborative roles in multidisciplinary teams.
Approach to supervision	• Supervision in student-led clinics needs to be flexible and adaptable to student competency and stage of learning, ranging from observation to autonomous practice, ensuring both safety and effective skill development. • Supervision includes role modelling, reflective practice and peer learning – especially in interprofessional contexts – to foster collaboration, self-assessment and a deeper understanding of team-based care.
Mode of delivery	• Three models of student-led clinics include university-affiliated, community-based and hybrid, each offering unique benefits for student learning and community engagement. • Governance and quality assurance are essential in all models to ensure safe, ethical practice under the supervision of registered professionals. • Mode of delivery (online or face to face) should align with community needs and clinic goals, ensuring accessibility and relevance.
Planning and preparation	• Establishing a student-led clinic requires identifying a service gap, engaging stakeholders and addressing regulatory, ethical and logistical needs, including governance, supervision and infrastructure.

Table 11.1 continued

	• Clinic processes such as referral pathways, confidentiality, record keeping and outcome measures must be clearly defined, alongside marketing, quality assurance and complaint procedures. • Pre-placement training for educators and students is essential, covering clinic structure, supervision models, interprofessional collaboration and practical readiness.
Implementing placement	• Implementing a student-led clinic needs a structured, phased approach with strong governance, operational readiness and a focus on sustainability and patient-centred care. • Comprehensive student preparation – including training, role play and clear orientation – builds confidence and sets clear expectations for clinical practice. • Ongoing supervision, peer learning, emotional support and continuous feedback promote skill development, wellbeing and professional growth.
Post-placement	• Post-placement evaluation of student-led clinics should include feedback from students, practice educators and service users to assess learning outcomes, patient satisfaction and service effectiveness, helping improve future placements and secure funding for sustainability.

clinical skills, including assessment, diagnosis and treatment planning. This real-world exposure fosters critical thinking and decision-making abilities in a controlled, supervised environment. Furthermore, students can learn to perform under pressure, develop confidence and increase competence in their clinical practice (Jones et al., 2018).

- **Promoting interprofessional collaboration**: Allied health practice frequently requires collaboration across multiple healthcare professions. Student-led clinics provide a unique setting where students from various disciplines can work together, simulating an interprofessional healthcare team. This collaborative experience not only promotes communication and teamwork but also prepares students for future interprofessional practice, which is vital in improving patient care outcomes.
- **Developing professionalism and ethical practices**: In addition to clinical competencies, student-led clinics offer a platform for students to refine their professionalism and ethical decision-making. These settings promote the development of empathy, confidentiality, cultural sensitivity and ethical conduct, all of which are essential competencies for future practitioners (Sick et al., 2017;

Abrey et al., 2022). Students can learn about patient-centred care, ensuring their practice aligns with the core values of respect, autonomy and beneficence.

- **Improving reflective practice and self-assessment**: As students engage with real patients in a supervised environment, they are encouraged to reflect on their experiences, identify areas for improvement and assess their professional growth. Such reflective practices are key to becoming a self-directed learner – a fundamental aspect of lifelong professional development. Feedback from patients, supervisors and peers further enhances this process, ensuring continuous improvement in clinical practice.

This suggests that the potential learning can be broad for students and therefore specific clinics can be set up to provide more emphasis on discrete areas of learning, e.g., interprofessional working or developing professional reasoning. As student-led clinics are developed with student learning at their heart, they can be designed in such a way that their learning outcomes are integral to the design, which is a real strength of this approach. The student-led clinic can be integrated into the curriculum to provide hands-on experience or offered as a placement choice within a programme of study. A further strength of the approach is that a student-led clinic can be set up to meet a service gap in the community offering a service to meet unmet needs for groups and communities to improve health and wellbeing whilst benefiting student learning (Goodfellow et al., 2017). This can be advantageous for higher education institutions, as a student-led clinic may support them to meet their altruistic and charitable contributions within their local communities aligned to their vision or mission statements. On balance, the student-led clinics affords beneficial outcomes for learners, service users and higher education institutions.

Approach to supervision with student-led clinics

The support and supervision of students participating in a student-led clinic is an integral part of the planning and operation of the clinic. The role of a practice educator is to support and guide students to ensure that they are consulting with service users in a manner that is both effective and safe, while also creating an environment for learning that prepares students for practice (Abrey et al., 2022). Within a student-led clinic, the design and setup of the clinic will determine who the supervisor is; this can be a member of the faculty team from the university or a qualified healthcare profession funded to provide supervision. This will be determined by the resourcing and funding arrangements of the student-led clinic. The practice educator may adopt several strategies for providing supervision and support. These can include role modelling of clinical skills to gather information, assessments and interventions, and case study discussions, while being supervised in interprofessional groups and engaging in reflection on their experiences and learning (Hu et al., 2018). The level of supervision and support will be determined by the learner's stage of the programme and competency displayed aligned to the intended learning outcomes of the placement; this can range from observation to autonomous practice with varying degrees of observation and support from the practice educator aligned to the learning needs. A challenge, in terms of supervising groups of students within a student-led clinic environment, can be providing a balance between enabling students to engage in clinical activities while also providing an appropriate level of supervision to ensure safe practice (Maple et al., 2023). As most student-led clinics have peer learning, supervisory structures need to account for this (see Chapter 4), because this often occurs in the context of interprofessional learning – then it is important to ensure students have opportunities for developing self-reflection and appraisal, and peer feedback. Learning with an interprofessional and team working focus is integral to learning in this context (Hopkins et al., 2022).

Mode of delivery of student-led clinics

In terms of mode of delivery in the design of a student-led clinic, you need to first decide the structure and model of the student-led clinic. This includes consideration of quality and governance arrangements. The main types of student-led clinics include the following.

- **University-affiliated student-led clinics**: These operate within the university setting (normally health sciences faculties or university hospitals) and are supervised by university staff who are professionally registered. The clinic is usually integrated into the academic curriculum to provide opportunities for hands-on learning. The benefits of being based in university is the close alignment this can have with intended learning outcomes, as this can be controlled and directed by university staff.
- **Community-based student-led clinics**: These tend to be run in local communities, often working with underserved or marginalised populations. These community-based clinics are often run in partnership with non-profit, public health organisations, charities or independent services. They tend to provide free or low-cost services to address health inequalities or unmet needs of local communities or groups. The benefit of this model is to provide a service in a real-world setting that promotes community engagement and social responsibility.
- **Hybrid model of student-led clinics**: These combine university-affiliated and community-based models. They offer both on-campus and off-campus placement experiences. This provides opportunity for flexible learning whilst

addressing community health needs. This model provides more structure and direction from the university to direct support the learning opportunities. This joint model offers chance for interprofessional collaboration and can be a sustainable model by combining university funding and community resources.

In setting up any of these models of student-led clinics, there needs to be consideration of the funding, governance and quality assurance arrangements to ensure that learners and service users are supported. The student-led clinics need appropriate oversight by registered healthcare professionals to ensure that they adhere to expected clinical and ethical standards. The mode of delivery, whether online or face to face, should be designed to best meet the needs of the intended community or group accessing the clinic.

Planning and preparation for student-led clinics

Initially when setting up a student-led clinic, you need to ensure that you have a clear population with which to work. This requires identification of a gap in service provision which the student-led clinic could meet. Stakeholder engagement is needed to ensure that collaboration and partnership arrangements between university, community partners and potential funding sources makes sense. Planning should be cognisant of any regulatory or legal considerations, e.g., insurance and ethical; all professional and ethical practices must been in place before the student-led clinic starts operating. Once the focus of the service is defined, and the model of student-led (e.g., university-affiliated or community-based) clinic agreed, then the physical infrastructure, scope of the service, governance and leadership structures need to be defined and established. This includes considering the location and physical resource requirements of the service, the scale of the offering, the frequency of the clinic, the types of appointments to be offered, the level of space or technology required and the personnel requirements needed, e.g., who will supervise and lead the service, as well as providing all the necessary coordination and support needed for the student placements.

As the student-led clinic is delivering a health service, the processes of the clinic would also need to be defined in terms of referral points, length of service on offer and onward referral routes if required. This also requires some public awareness raising and marketing to advertise the clinic. Additionally, quality procedures, service-user feedback and relevant outcome measures need to be considered to reflective the service focus and measure impact. Also, procedures for raising concerns and complaints would need to be developed to ensure that service users have a process to express their opinions. Record keeping, documentation, data protection – including any information technology resources and support – and confidentiality issues must be considered and relevant procedures put in place. There may also be implications for training of staff and learners.

Once these elements of setting up a student-led clinic are established, planning is necessary for training and pre-placement preparation required for practice educators and learners. Practice educators need to be familiar and comfortable with the structure and intended services to provide relevant professional support to learners. They also need to be confident with the planned model of supervision and – in most cases – peer learning that is typically a core part of the structure of student-led clinics. Learners require an induction to the placement and awareness of the focus, setup and procedures of the student-led clinic. Given the typical interprofessional focus of student-led clinics, pre-placement preparation could also focus on identifying the readiness of students in terms of being able to deal with and address potential negative attitudes to interprofessional working (Shrader et al., 2010).

Implementation of student-led clinics

Successfully implementing a student-led clinic requires a clear governance structure, operational readiness and continuous quality improvement. It needs to be a structured and phased approach, ensuring sustainability, compliance and educational benefits. By focusing on patient-centred care, student education and sustainability, a student-led clinic can make a lasting impact on both healthcare training and community service. The initial phase of a student-led clinic requires a comprehensive approach to training and orientation; this can include training about processes and expectations, e.g., procedures and documentation, but can also focus on simulation or role playing of patient interactions expected in setting to build confidence and student expectations.

During placement, a comprehensive approach also needs to be taken to supervision and mentorship. This includes their allocated practice educator but can also take form of peer mentorship whereby students learn with and from each other within structured clinical tasks or allocated work. As a practice educator, you should encourage a collaborative working environment that is supportive and creates safe space for students to learn together. The unique setup of a student-led clinic may require consideration of supporting students to manage their wellbeing and stress levels, as well as ensuring the development of professional socialisation and identity within the student-led clinic. Throughout placement there should be clear structure for formal and informal feedback to ensure ongoing development and clear action plan and expectation of learning between the student and the practice educator, including regular performance reviews and reflection on learning and future actions. Supporting students in a student-led clinic requires a comprehensive approach that integrates training, mentorship, emotional wellbeing, academic development and continuous feedback. By fostering a supportive and structured environment, students can enhance their clinical skills, gain confidence and contribute effectively to patient care.

Post-placement for student-led clinics

A post-placement evaluation ensures that student-led clinics provide meaningful learning experiences and quality patient care. Post-placement evaluation should consider student achievement of intended learning outcomes and feedback on their experience, as well as considering service-user feedback on their use of the service either through patient satisfaction survey or outcome measures. Tokolahi et al. (2021) suggested the measurement of outcomes of service delivery could be a helpful strategy to secure funding. By incorporating students, practice educators and patient feedback, the clinic can continuously evolve to better support future healthcare professionals and provide evidence for funding to support a sustainable student-led clinic.

PRACTICE EXAMPLES

Example 1 – University of South Australia (USA): USA operates several community clinics that are open to the public, providing quality, accessible and cost-effective services. A range of clinics operate which are either student-run or led by a qualified clinician with students being involved in the facilitation of service delivery. One clinic in operation is an occupational therapy clinic for children and youth; a qualified clinician is present all year round to support continuity of care and case load management with students being involved in a range of clinic and service development tasks, including planning and implementation of clinic-based sessions and resource development. The clinic is in a city-based campus and offers students the opportunity for interprofessional working with other co-located clinics such as physiotherapy, exercise physiology, podiatry and speech pathology. There are also general practice and nursing clinics on site. The clinic runs five days a week with students participating in approximately four patient sessions a day. Students are supervised by a qualified clinician, and the clinic provides opportunities for peer learning and supervision.

Example 2 – Glasgow Caledonian University (GCU) student-led vision clinic (orthoptics): GCU operates a large vision centre on site, based on the ground floor of the Govan Mbeki Building and open to students and staff of the university, as well as the public. Services include optometry and orthoptics. For the purposes of this case study, we will focus on the orthoptics component.

The student-led orthoptics clinic runs two afternoons per week, staffed by fourth-year orthoptics students and fourth-year optometry students. The orthoptic students lead, focusing specifically on binocular vision disorders, which is a specialty of the teaching team. Patients can be babies, children, adults and older adults. The clinic is free, with the teaching team acting as highly trained professionals offering a student-led service. It serves to work alongside NHS provision, both working in harmony with NHS orthoptics services, and/or taking the pressure of NHS services by providing an alternative. If a patient requires urgent referral, this is done by the clinic. Students never work alone, and the supervisor must be able to discuss and explain any action they take. Patients can self-refer or be referred by optometrists, general practitioners, etc. The most common routes to the clinic are via optometry referral and self-referral. However, the clinic has noted an increase in self-referral via social media raising awareness of binocular vision disorders.

It runs in addition to placement hours required of the students. Students work in pairs, threes or fours, making maximal use of the benefits of peer learning, including near-peer learning, and serving to increase the level of knowledge, understanding and respect between the professions of optometry and orthoptics. Additional benefits include creating a database of patients which can then also be used in simulations, and for patient consultation activities such as programme reviews. The clinic is also able to offer CPD opportunities to practicing orthoptists and provides a place where the power and benefits of peer learning can be shown, as well as how to operationalise these in a space which may be space and resource tight.

Every patient is offered two hours of clinic time, and in each cubical (3 × 3m) is the patient, who may have a carer/guardian with them, four students and one supervisor, who would usually pop in and out. For the students, the afternoon session involved a briefing, total immersion in their one service user for a two-hour period, then a debrief, which focuses on discussion and exploration of the full patient journey.

Challenges include the need for more supervisors. The clinic would like to include practicing orthoptists/practice educator orthoptists as supervisors, coming in for just one afternoon to benefit from the CPD experience and model new methods of practice-based learning. Benefits include the resultant wide external networking the clinic has provided. Additionally, with the removal of the time pressure component that exists in NHS and private services, student learning is optimised.

Example 3 – Haven for Hope (Geelhoed et al., 2019): This involves physiotherapy learners at University of Texas Health in San Antonio (UTHSA) in the United States working in the provision of a student-run free clinic offering pro bono physiotherapy services at a homelessness shelter. Learners can treat patients under the direct supervision of licensed physiotherapists, and the clinic is held once per month.

> *Referrals come from the onsite physician and nurse practitioner, as well as a separate SRFC [student-run free clinic] run by the School of Medicine of UTHSA. Each cohort of DPT [doctorate of physical therapy] students has a representative in charge of organizing volunteers, coordinating supervision, and facilitating transportation. Students typically volunteer for a 4-hour shift and as a group see about 5–15 patients every month.*
>
> (Geelhoed et al., 2019, p. 221)

Example 4 – Indiana University Student Outreach Clinic (George et al., 2017): This is a pro bono, community-based, interprofessional student-led clinic which is dedicated to the removal of healthcare barriers. The student-led clinic provides a range of learning opportunities which include "clinical competency, professional values, civic engagement, interprofessional education and collaborative practice (IPECP), peer mentorship, and leadership development" (George et al., 2017, p. 54). The mission of the student outreach clinic is:

> to provide medically underserved and uninsured populations within Indiana communities with access to free health care while providing students from multiple disciplines opportunity for professional development. Its primary goal is to decrease health care inequality.
>
> (George et al., 2017, p. 54)

SUMMING UP WITH KEY PRINCIPLES AND FUTURE DIRECTIONS

The evidence for student-led clinics is nascent but it suggests that they can provide an invaluable learning opportunity for learners, as well as serve local communities. However, several challenges have been outlined in relation to the delivery of student-led clinics including funding, planning, time pressures and the diversity of the patient population. Moving forward, key areas to consider for education providers in developing this model of practice-based learning include effective planning of operational aspects of a clinic, aligning the curriculum in order to ensure the student-led clinics provides "consistent and sustainable interprofessional learning opportunities" and establishing a clear vision in terms of focus and objectives (Tokolahi et al., 2021).

REFERENCES

Abrey, C., De Silva, N., Godwin, J., Jacotine, T., Raab, D., Urquhart, K., Mumford, K., McLaughlin, P. and Vaughan, B. (2022). Does the student-led osteopathy clinical learning environment prepare students for practice? *BMC Medical Education*, *22*(603), pp. 1–9. https://doi.org/10.1186/s12909-022-03658-3

Beveridge, J. and Pentland, D. (2020). A mapping review of models of practice education in allied health and social care professions. *British Journal of Occupational Therapy*, *83*(8), pp. 488–513.

Briggs, L. and Fronek, P. (2020). Student experiences and perceptions of participation in student-led health clinics: A systematic review. *Journal of Social Work Education*, *56*(2), pp. 238–259. https://doi.org/10.1080/10437797.2019.1656575

Chartered Society of Physiotherapy. (2023). *Principles of practice – based learning*. Available at: https://www.csp.org.uk/publications/ahp-principles-practice-based-learning (Accessed 24 April 2024).

Geelhoed, M. A., Callaway, S. M., Cruz, J. M. and Subramanian, S. K. (2019). Attitudes of physical therapy students toward the population currently experiencing homelessness. A pilot study. *Journal of Allied Health*, *48*(3), pp. 220–225.

George, L., Bemenderfer, S., Cappel, M., Goncalves, K., Hornstein, M., Savage, C., Altenburger, P., Bellew, J. and Loghmani, T. (2017). A model for providing free patient care and integrating student learning and professional development in an interprofessional student-led clinic. *Journal of Physical Therapy Education*, *31*(2), pp. 54–66.

Gillies, J., Bishop, M., McGehee, W., Lulofs-MacPherson, K. and Dunleavy, K. (2019). Impact on clinical performance of required participation a student-run pro bono clinic. *Journal of Physical Therapy Education*, *33*(3), pp. 209–214.

Goodfellow, L. M., Jones, P. and Smith, H. (2017). Addressing health inequities through student-led clinics in community settings. *Journal of Health Promotion*, *39*(3), pp. 241–252.

Gustafsson, L., Hutchinson, L., Theodoros, D., Williams, K., Copley, A., Fagan, A. and Desha, L. (2016). Healthcare students' experiences of an interprofessional, student-led neuro-rehabilitation community-based clinic. *Journal of Interprofessional Care*, *30*(2), pp. 259–261. https://doi.org/10.3109/13561820.2015.1086730

Haines, T. P., Kent, F. and Keating, J. L. (2014). Interprofessional student clinics: An economic evaluation of collaborative clinical placement education. *Journal of Interprofessional Care*, *28*(4), pp. 292–298. https://doi.org/10.3109/13561820.2013.874983

Hopkins, S., Bacon, R. and Flynn, A. (2022). Student outcomes for interprofessional education in student led clinics: A rapid review. *Journal of Interprofessional Care*, *36*(2), pp. 234–244.

Hu, T., Cox, K. A. and Nyhof-Young, J. (2018). Investigating student perceptions at an interprofessional student-run free clinic serving marginalised populations. *Journal of Interprofessional Care*, *32*(1), pp. 75–79. https://doi.org/10.1080/13561820.2017.1363724

Interprofessional Education Collaborative IPEC. (2023). *IPEC core competencies for interprofessional collaborative practice: Version 3*. Available at: IPEC core competencies for interprofessional collaborative practice: Version 3. ipecollaborative.org. (Accessed 1 July 2024).

Jones, M., Roberts, S. and Clarke, A. (2018). The role of student-led clinics in developing clinical confidence and competence: A systematic review. *Clinical Teacher*, *16*(4), pp. 309–314.

Kavanagh, J., Kearns, A. and McGarry, T. (2015). The benefits and challenges of student-led clinics within an Irish context. *Journal of Practice Teaching and Learning*, *13*(2–3), pp. 58–72.

Kent, F., Martin, N. and Keating, J. (2016). Interprofessional student-led clinics: An innovative approach to the support of older people in the community. *Journal of Interprofessional Care*, 30(1), pp. 123–128. https://doi.org/10.3109/13561820.2015.1070133

Maple, M., O'Neill, K., Gartshore, S., Clark, J., White, J. and Pearce, T. (2023). School-based multidisciplinary student-led clinics in health and Australian accreditation standards: A scoping review. *Australian Journal Rural Health*, *31*, pp. 1168–1183. https://doi.org/10.1111/ajr.13051

Passmore, A., Persic, C., Countryman, D., Rankine, L., Henderson, M., Hu, T., Nyhof-Young, J. and Cott, C. (2016). Student and preceptor experiences at an inter-professional student-run clinic: A physical therapy perspective. *Physiotherapy Canada*, *68*(4), pp. 391–397.

Schutte, T., Tichelaar, J., Dekker, R. S., Agtmael, M. A., Vries, T. P. and Richir, M. C. (2015). Learning in student-run clinics: A systematic review. *Medical Education*, *49*(3), pp. 249–263.

Schutte, T., Tichelaar, J., Donker, E., Richir, M. C., Westerman, M. and Van Agtmael, M. A. (2018). Clarifying learning experiences in student-run clinics: A qualitative study. *BMC Medical Education*, *18*, p. 244.

Shrader, S., Thompson, A. and Gonsalves, W. (2010). Assessing Student Attitudes as a Result of Participating in an Interprofessional Healthcare Elective Associated with a Student-Run Free Clinic. *Journal of Research in Interprofessional Practice and Education*, *1*(3), pp. 281–230.

Sick, B., Zhang, L. and Weber-Main, A. M. (2017). Changes in health professional students' attitudes toward the underserved. Impact of extended participation in an interprofessional student-run free clinic. *Journal of Allied Health*, *46*(4), pp. 213–219.

Simpson, S. A. and Long, J. (2007). Medical student-run health clinics: Important contributors to patient care and medical education. *Society of General Internal Medicine*, *22*(3), pp. 352–356.

Tokolahi, E., Broman, P., Longhurst, G., Pearce, A., Cook, C., Andersen, P. and Brownie, S. (2021). Student-led clinics in Aotearoa New Zealand: A scoping review with stakeholder consultation. *Journal of Multidisciplinary Healthcare*, *14*, pp. 2053–2066.

Walpola, R. L. and Schneider, C. R. (2018). Longitudinal interprofessional student-led clinics – a formula for implementation. *International Journal of Pharmacy Practice*, *26*, pp. 473–474. https://doi.org/10.1111/ijpp.12495

Wynne, D. and Cooper, K. (2019). Student led physical rehabilitation groups and clinics in entry-level health education: A scoping review protocol. *JBI Database of Systematic Reviews and Implementation Reports*, *17*(6), pp. 1092–1100. https://doi.org/10.11124/JBISRIR-2017-003990

Wynne, D. and Cooper, K. (2021). Student led physical rehabilitation groups and clinics in entry-level health education: A scoping review. *JBI Evidence Synthesis*, *19*(11), pp. 2958–2992. https://doi.org/10.11124/JBIES-20-00340

Yap, J., Broman, P., Andersen, P. and Brownie, S. (2024). Learning by doing: Students' experiences of interprofessional education and community partnership in a pilot student-run clinic. A practice report. *Student Success*, *15*(1), pp. 122–129.

Chapter 12

Public health and community-based rehabilitation

Community-based practice placement models for social transformation

Roshan Galvaan, Liesl Peters, Isaac Amanquarnor, Lisa Forrest and Anita Volkert

CHAPTER OVERVIEW

Health and rehabilitation professions are increasingly recognising how their professions can contribute to addressing the social determinants of health. When these perspectives are included into curricula, it involves a public health perspective and justice orientation to practice whereby students can contribute to social transformation. This chapter will draw on public health and justice-oriented theories to describe key principles for creating community-based placements. The application of these principles in the design of the placements is elucidated concerning essential features of building partnerships with placement sites and applying a critical approach to practice. This is illustrated through referring to a practice demonstration site in South Africa and a case study of how students are prepared for community-based placements in Scotland.

CHAPTER OBJECTIVES

- To describe supporting theories that undergird community-based practice placements.
- To share essential elements that should be considered when designing community-based placement models.
- To provide examples that can be used to enhance an understanding of how a community-based practice model evolves and insight into how teaching and learning might occur as we prepare students to engage in this kind of placement.

DOI: 10.4324/9781003411765-12

OVERVIEW

This chapter outlines community-based placement practice models, which foreground public health, community development and a justice orientation to practice. It begins by outlining the rationale for these models and then describes supporting evidence for their application. Thereafter, the key features that may be used for designing community-based placements are described. Finally, examples of applying these models of practice are provided.

THE NEED FOR COMMUNITY-BASED PLACEMENT MODELS

A biomedical lens of health has dominated the healthcare paradigm, shaping the perspectives of various health and social care professions, including occupational therapy. While valuable in understanding and treating specific diseases and impairments, it offers a reductionist view that often oversimplifies the complex interplay of social, economic and political factors that influence the wellbeing of individuals and populations. It tends to isolate health issues from their broader context, focusing on individual responsibility for health while neglecting the crucial influence of socioeconomic disparities, cultural dynamics and systemic inequalities on health and wellbeing (Kapilashrami et al., 2015).

Over the last 30 years, approaches to practice in occupational therapy and occupational therapy education have evolved to incorporate a more inclusive view that recognises the social and political determinants of health and aims to equip students with the skills to navigate these complex influences through practice placement learning opportunities (Golos and Tekuzener, 2021; Mattila, 2019; Richards and Galvaan, 2018). A public health perspective of human occupation foregrounds that underlying structural factors create institutions and policies that govern participation and influence health (Wilcock, 1998).

Adopting a public health perspective involves appreciating how structural conditions within countries and globally shape opportunities for and patterns of participation in occupation. It recognises that public policies and the structure and function of institutions orchestrate invisible social rules that govern social interaction and participation in occupations. The combined influence of these policies and rules across different systems may give rise to inequitable opportunities for participation. Common examples are how a person's nationality or citizenship status may influence the types of activities that they have access to or the spaces where they experience a sense of belonging, or how local regulations limit which school children may have access to. An awareness of these inequities could lead to identifying ways in which workplaces could recognise the value that different worker roles add to the workforce within different organisations – or occupational therapists or other allied health professionals could identify possibilities for contributing to advocacy initiatives and lobbying for policy changes. Therefore, a public health perspective invites occupational therapists and other allied health professionals to analyse how institutions may create conditions that lead to inequitable opportunities for participation. This matters since such inequitable opportunities create the risk of forms of occupational injustice – and therefore negative consequences on health and wellbeing (Stadnyk et al., 2010).

While occupational therapy students in many programmes may be placed in communities as they complete the practice placements as a requirement for their qualifications, the focus may often be on providing medical rehabilitation to individuals, rather than responding to issues of inequity and injustice made apparent through applying community development or public health perspectives to practice. In this chapter, we use the term 'community-based placements' to describe sites of occupational therapy practice that embrace these public health perspectives and community development approaches to contribute to equity and justice through student practice. Community-based placements involve learning opportunities to address underlying, systemic factors influencing health and wellbeing. At the same time, students are placed in a community rather than in a hospital or health service setting. Students learn from and with community members, often drawing on participatory processes while providing services that benefit communities. This type of practice is referred to as community development practice (CDP), referring to services and approaches that allow students to engage with all the realities of everyday life with which community members deal.

The vocabularies and epistemologies of CDP can be interpreted in multiple ways, dependent on local needs and priorities for occupational therapy practice in different global contexts (Hyett et al., 2023). This means that different practice frameworks might be drawn upon in different contexts to support this kind of work. These frameworks, for instance, include – but are not limited to – 'social occupational therapy', 'Occupation-based Community Development' (ObCD); the 'Canadian Community Development Practice Process', 'Decolonising person-centred care approaches' and the 'Community Centered Practice Framework' (Hyett et al., 2023). The Participatory Occupational Justice Framework (POJF) has also been proposed as relevant for practitioners needing to centre issues of equity and justice in their work (Townsend and Whiteford, 2005). When used to support the education of occupational therapy students, these frameworks and approaches are designed to impart students with essential knowledge and skill sets aimed at partnering with communities to address the social and political determinants of health and their imposed limitations on occupational engagement/everyday life. The practice at community-based placements addresses the multifaceted health challenges confronting communities, including socioeconomic, sociopolitical and health disparities. Community-based placement models must, therefore, engage theories and frameworks for CDP, as well as principles for role-emerging occupational therapy.

In the UK, many universities have incorporated role-emerging placement (REP) models as a strategy to afford students community-based placement opportunities within health and social care settings that lack established occupational therapy roles (Clarke et al., 2014). Like the CDP model, the REP model involves students being supervised by off-site placement supervisors. This placement framework is intentionally structured to equip students with essential skills pertinent to their prospective professional practice within the dynamic landscape of contemporary health and social care. Emphasis is placed on promoting health and overall wellbeing while addressing healthcare disparities (Clarke et al., 2014). The REP approach is crucial in bridging the gap between traditional clinical settings and the evolving demands of healthcare practices (Clarke et al., 2014; Golos and Tekuzener, 2021). By immersing students in environments where occupational therapy roles are not predefined, this pedagogical strategy aims to cultivate adaptability, critical thinking and innovative problem-solving skills among aspiring occupational therapists.

Community-based placements adopting a community development approach aim to equip students with the necessary skills to work in socially transformative ways. In this chapter, we describe how we have used the ObCD and the POJF frameworks as theoretical support for occupational therapy practices that contribute to justice and equity in community-based placement settings.

COMMUNITY-BASED PLACEMENT MODELS AND THEIR CONTRIBUTION TO STUDENT LEARNING

Like conventional placement models, community-based placement models provide students with a valuable chance to make links between theories and practice. In contrast to occupational therapy role–established placement settings, community-based placement settings often have no predefined occupational therapy role or mentor figure on site. Students are assigned off-site supervisors who facilitate their learning experiences at placement settings. Through community-based placements, students become equipped to engage with issues of social transformation. The way that these placements are designed are integral to facilitating learning.

Community-based placements should ideally be created by applying the following four essential principles.

1. They should involve identifying practice sites that require critical occupational therapy services and could benefit from this contribution. That is, services that engage with unjust conditions shaping people's lives and their related occupational engagement (Hammell and Iwama, 2012).
2. They should offer flexibility in defining and developing the occupational therapist's role so that relevant and emergent needs can be responded to and worked with.
3. They should prioritise the partnerships between educators, students and site partners.
4. They should foster and empower students in cultivating the essential competencies required for effectively grappling with issues related to the social and political determinants of health.

In placements applying these principles, students learn various skills and competencies focused on health promotion, wellness, human rights and social justice (Mattila, 2019; Richards and Galvaan, 2018; Golos and Tekuzener, 2021; Krenzer, 2019). Our experiences of developing and facilitating community-based placements are rooted in co-creating and using the ObCD framework (Galvaan and Peters, 2017a) and the POJF (Whiteford and Townsend, 2011). Authors Galvaan and Peters are co-creators of ObCD, and Amanquarnor and Forrest have used this framework in their teaching. All authors have made use of the POJF in the teaching and service-learning arenas within their diverse higher education contexts.

Brief descriptions of the ObCD and POJF

The ObCD framework serves as a guide for practice in community development, integrating philosophies and theories from community development, organisational learning and development, critical occupational therapy and occupational science (Galvaan and Peters, 2017a, 2017b). Its development was motivated by a commitment to resisting hegemony and fostering social change among marginalised and disadvantaged populations, thereby countering societal injustices and oppression (Galvaan and Peters, 2017a, 2017b). The overarching goal is to promote social inclusion and challenge the systemic and environmental conditions that limit participation, especially for marginalised populations. In community-based practice placements, the ObCD framework is a thinking tool that empowers students to collaboratively design campaigns with marginalised groups to address specific community needs (Richards and Galvaan, 2018). The ObCD framework has assisted student practice in South Africa, where communities are marked by the historical legacies of colonisation and apartheid (Krenzer, 2019).

Similarly, the POJF was developed as a non-linear analytic and pragmatic framework to interrogate and respond to the evident occupational justices in context, together with communities (Whiteford and Townsend, 2011). Programmes and services are devised in response to injustices, mobilising and coordinating necessary resources (Townsend and Whiteford, 2005). The end goal is to mitigate occupational injustices through centring occupation and client-centredness as tools for change (Townsend and Whiteford, 2005).

DESIGN FEATURES OF A COMMUNITY-BASED PLACEMENT

The four principles that underscore a community-based placement also direct their design. These principles seek to enact a mutually beneficial relationship for students, the institution/organisation where students are placed and the higher learning institution placing students. This section describes the design features related to building such partnerships and promulgating an innovative, critical approach to practice.

Community-based placements create potential opportunities for innovative practices beyond rigidly defined practice models, leveraging the chance to collaborate with site partners in defining the potential contribution that students make at the practice placement. This involves innovation rather than only the application of knowledge and practice. Also, instead of a firm idea of what the contribution might entail, a collaborative exploration occurs which conscientiously centres a critical occupational perspective in practice. This means paying attention to how this partnership is constructed and maintained longitudinally as part of designing the community-based placement.

Christie (2018) suggests that the notion of partnership often holds a generic meaning, although it can manifest in various nuanced ways. The construct of forming a partnership may have different meanings for different people and is constituted across structural and social differences (Christie, 2018). In creating partnerships that support community-based placements, it becomes necessary to nurture an ethics of engagement that is alert to the asymmetries that could exist in such partnerships (Christie, 2018). Institutions of higher learning often have significant power in communities. As such, we have a moral imperative to ensure that this power is exercised in ways that open a pathway through which mutual benefit and growth is possible for the institution and community-based organisations. The voice of the organisation/community should be foregrounded in this partnership.

The notion of building relationships – as a crucial part of initiation within the ObCD process – supports the development of mutually beneficial partnerships (Galvaan and Peters, 2017a, 2017b). A concerted effort towards investing in relationships that can support practice occurs through negotiating the community-based practice site at the outset and allowing for the evolution of practice at the site during the student placement. As part of building relationships in the initiation phase of the ObCD framework, students/practitioners are prompted to consider their intersectional social positions and those of others with whom they work during the placement. Critical questions are proposed to support this process, such as the following.

- How does your intersectional identity influence the way you develop under-standing and build relationships in this context?
- How does your identity as part of a prestigious university and profession influ-ence your relationships and what privileges you may have?
- What strategies may you apply to prepare and allow yourself to engage authentically and equally in this context?

(Galvaan and Peters, 2013)

Relationship changes over time can be a marker of development (Taylor, 2000) and are reflected in how power is operationalised within these relationships. This means that when sites resist any impositions that the relationship brings, we see this as a strength and a sign of development within the partnership. This often manifests in the people at the community-based placement site beginning to increasingly signal how the placement should evolve. This is celebrated because it shows shifts as an outcome of implementing participatory approaches in our practices. It also means that it paves the way for a compelling collaborative exploration that can support an innovative occupational therapy service.

A critical occupational perspective seeks to unlock an understanding of the hegemonic aspects that keep marginalising contexts in place and certain social groups trapped in ways of doing that do not serve their health and wellbeing. Such an understanding grows over time and is supported through the mutually beneficial partnership described above. Since 2000, authors Galvaan and Peters have been developing a community-based practice demonstration site known as Facing Up. Students participate in this practice demonstration site as part of their BSc occupational therapy curriculum. Facing Up evolved through work with primary schools in an impoverished community on the Cape Flats[1] in Cape Town, South Africa. Using the design principles previously described, Facing Up has become a model for community-based practice placements and its blueprint has been used to guide the development of practice-based placements with other population groups in diverse settings across the Cape Town metropole. For examples of the kinds of work students at Facing Up are involved in, see www.facingup.uct.ac.za.

TEACHING AND LEARNING APPROACHES FOR PREPARING STUDENTS TO ENGAGE IN COMMUNITY-BASED PRACTICE PLACEMENTS

Since community-based practice placements require a focus on justice and equity and demand innovation, students need to be prepared to engage in such placements in their curricula. Depending on how CDP is taught at different tertiary institutions and in different global spaces, this could involve diverse vocabularies and practice models, as suggested earlier in this chapter. In our experience, we have found that utilising practice frameworks that push students to consider the critical implications of context on occupational engagement and the need to develop practice approaches that allow occupational therapists to better engage with issues of justice and equity can be helpful. In what follows, Forrest describes how she prepares students for this kind of practice placement.

Practice example at Glasgow Caledonian University

At Glasgow Caledonian University, the MSc (pre-registration) occupational therapy students undertake the module 'Occupational Justice, Policy and Societal Transformation' as part of their programme. This capstone module is in the final trimester of the two-year programme. A prime concern of occupational therapy is both inclusion and justice, addressing restrictions placed on individuals, groups or societies due to disability, poverty, violence or environmental disasters (Hocking and Townsend, 2015).

The module aims to build on students' knowledge of occupational therapy and broaden their critical thinking by prompting them to consider wider societal

---

1   The Cape Flats is a geographic area in Cape Town, South Africa, where people designated as Coloured and Black were forcibly removed during the implementation of the racial segregation laws under apartheid. More information about forced removals and apartheid legislation is available at: https://www.districtsix.co.za/about-district-six/

impact of occupation to achieve societal transformation and social justice. An evaluation of local and international policy is central to learning on the module that facilitates the micro, meso and macro perspectives, therefore supporting the student to actively engage as a global citizen. Overall, the learning on the module aims to equip the students with the knowledge, understanding and skills required to address restrictions placed on individuals, groups and societies due to disability, poverty, violence and environmental disasters (Hocking and Townsend, 2015).

Students are enabled to evaluate occupational justice for individuals, groups and societies both locally and globally. This is achieved by engaging in critical evaluation of contemporary global issues such as displaced individuals, climate justice and health promotion. In addition, learners are encouraged to critically evaluate the systemic, structural and societal influences of local and global contexts of these contemporary issues. Theories of occupational and social justice, social leadership, transformation and entrepreneurialism are explored to support the student to apply their knowledge of occupation to achieve sustainable and globally oriented societal change and align with the university's Common Good curriculum.

The learning and teaching strategy utilised on the module to maximise understanding and application of key frameworks is Problem-Based Learning (PBL) (Jones, 2006). This approach requires active, self-directed learning which supports the development of the skills required for learning; therefore, learning results from the process of working towards the understanding of or resolution of a problem (Jones, 2006).

Working in groups, students are presented with a trigger or case study example from a variety of practice-based examples from both the Global North and South. In groups, students then identify what they need to know and construct a strategy to enable them to learn and apply skills to solve the problem. The frameworks used within the module include the POJF (Whiteford et al., 2018) and the ObCD framework (Galvaan and Peters, 2014). Throughout the module, groups are encouraged to explore and apply both frameworks to develop an occupation-based solution to the problem identified. Each group then presented to the class to guide discussion, learning and feedback.

Using the frameworks and considering the role of occupational therapy working with individuals, groups and communities, the module enabled creative ideas to support social transformation and a vision for future occupational therapy.

BENEFITS FOR STUDENTS THROUGH COMMUNITY-BASED PRACTICE PLACEMENTS

Through the courses that the authors of this chapter are involved in at their various institutional contexts, students are exposed to relevant knowledge crucial for this experiential learning endeavour. Learning about how to engage and then becoming involved in a community-based practice placement model not only equips students with requisite knowledge and skills but also furnishes them with a comprehensive philosophical and practical framework for engaging in impactful community development work (Richards and Galvaan, 2018; Krenzer, 2019).

For instance, reflecting on the value of the module that Forrest facilitates, students described that:

> *The course felt purposeful and I really appreciated how the lecturers put in the time and effort to get us to think outside of our own experiences and perspectives and imagine ways as a global citizen to make changes to improve real world issues such as resources for those with disability, mitigating loneliness and social isolation, and tackling the lingering and detrimental effects of poverty, racism, hunger, environmental damage, and violence. To learn, it is important for me to see that the lecturers are passionate about what they are teaching which really helps me to engage more with the material. I appreciated the lecturer's passion for the course and for the guidance when choosing and producing our ideas for a project.*

> *Creating the project really made me think about ways in which I could make meaningful impacts in my corner of the world once I return home. I was able to get in contact with two friends who are social workers who were excited about my idea of a social cafe for elderly people to mitigate loneliness and it really opened my eyes up to the possibility of affecting positive change in the world.*

Educational approaches that prepare students to engage in such practice experiences represents a substantive response to the distinctive needs of marginalised or disadvantage populations, providing students with a robust foundation for meaningful community development interventions in their future practice. In describing the benefits of these kinds of learning opportunities, Richards and Galvaan (2018) indicate that there can be a notable shift in the notions of students and mentors about the traditional role of occupational therapy in community-based settings. They argued that experiential placements in the community heightened students' awareness of macro-level factors influencing

212 New Practice-based Learning in the Allied Health Professions

people's daily lives, encouraging critical reflection on sociopolitical influences on health and wellbeing in various contexts. Golos and Tekuzener (2021) highlighted students' struggle in identifying resources for interventions and stressed the need to prepare staff members better to align expectations with the reality of student capabilities. Despite the challenges, students reported advancements in professional and personal skills after the placements, emphasising successful experiences and increased confidence in core skills (Golos and Tekuzener, 2021).

SUMMING UP WITH KEY PRINCIPLES

In summary, this chapter collectively underscores the impact of public health and community-based placement models on students' professional development, affirming their value in nurturing competent, adaptable, and reflective prospective occupational therapists positioned to serve the changing expansive healthcare needs. By addressing and collaborating with individuals, populations and marginalised groups in community settings, students gain a comprehensive understanding of the political and social determinants of health, but they also – importantly – have an opportunity to contribute meaningfully to development in a mutually beneficial partnership with organisations and communities. Community-based practice models, therefore, go beyond imparting skills and move towards providing a philosophical and practical foundation for meaningful and innovative interventions *with* communities. These community-based placement models provide an opportunity to shift occupational therapy education towards developing competence in addressing sociopolitical determinants and nurturing competencies that extend beyond clinical boundaries. Simultaneously, the opportunity to innovate and work with community needs, in context, offers mutual benefit for students and organisations/communities alike.

REFERENCES

Christie, P. (2018). Enlarged thinking and assymetrical reciprocity in an ethics of engagement: A reflection on university-school partnerships. In P. Silbert, R. Galvaan and J. Clark (Eds.), *Partnerships in Action: University-School-Community*. Cape Town: HSRC Press.

Clarke, C., Martin, M., Sadlo, G. and de Visser, R. (2014). The development of an authentic professional identity on role-emerging placements. *British Journal of Occupational Therapy*, *77*(5), pp. 222–229.

Galvaan, R. and Peters, L. (2013). *Open education resource: A strategy for occupation-based community development*. Available at: http://hdl.handle.net/11427/6651

Galvaan, R. and Peters, L. (2014). *Occupation based community development*. Available at: https://vula.uct.ac.za/access/content/group/9c29ba04-b1ee-49b9-8c85-9a468b556ce2/OBCDF/pages/intro.html

Galvaan, R. and Peters, L. (2017a). Occupation-based community development: Confronting the politics of occupation. In *Occupational Therapies without Borders: Integrating Justice with Practice* (pp. 283–291).

Galvaan, R. and Peters, L. (2017b). Occupation-based community development: A critical approach to occupational therapy. In S. Dsouza, R. Galvaan and E. Ramugondo (Eds.), *Concepts in Occupational Therapy: Understanding Southern Perspectives* (pp. 172–187). India: Manupal University Press.

Golos, A. and Tekuzener, E. (2021). Student and supervisor perspectives on the effectiveness of community-based placements for occupational therapy students. *BMC Medical Education*, 21, pp. 1–11.

Hammell, K. R. W. and Iwama, M. K. (2012). Well-being and occupational rights: An imperative for critical occupational therapy. *Scandinavian Journal of Occupational Therapy*, 19(5), pp. 385–394.

Hocking, C. and Townsend, E. (2015). Driving social change: Occupational therapists' contributions to occupational justice. *World Federation of Occupational Therapists Bulletin*, pp. 1–4.

Hyett, N., Peters, L., Gibson, C., Serrata Malfitano, A. P., Lauckner, H., Leclair, L. and Galvaan, R. (2023). International community of practice: Learning from experiences of community development and social occupational therapy. *Cadernos Brasileiros de Terapia Ocupacional*, 31, p. e3551.

Jones, R. W. (2006). Problem-based learning: Description, advantages, disadvantages, scenarios and facilitation. *Anaesth Intensive Care*, 34, pp. 485–488.

Kapilashrami, A., Hill, S. and Meer, N. (2015). What can health inequalities researchers learn from an intersectionality perspective? Understanding social dynamics with an inter-categorical approach? *Social Theory & Health*, 13, pp. 288–307.

Krenzer, M. L. M. (2019). *A case study exploring the application of the occupation-based community development framework: Co-constructing humanising praxis* (Master's thesis, Faculty of Health Sciences).

Mattila, A. (2019). Perceptions and outcomes of occupational therapy students participating in community engaged learning: A mixed-methods approach. *The Open Journal of Occupational Therapy*, 7(4), pp. 1–17.

Richards, L. A. and Galvaan, R. (2018). Developing a socially transformative focus in occupational therapy: Insights from South African practice. *South African Journal of Occupational Therapy*, 48(1), pp. 3–8.

Stadnyk, R. L., Townsend, E. A. and Wilcock, A. A. (2010). Occupational justice. In C. H. Christiansen and E. A. Townsend (Eds.), *Introduction to Occupation: The Art and Science of Living* (2nd ed., pp. 329–358). Pearson Education.

Taylor, J. (2000). *Organisations and Development: Towards Building a Practice*. Cape Town: Community Development Resource Association.

Townsend, E. and Whiteford, G. (2005). A participatory occupational justice framework. Population-based processes of practice. In F. Kronenberg, S. Simó Algado and N. Pollard (Eds.), *Occupational Therapy without Borders: Learning from the Spirit of Survivors*. Edinburgh: Churchill Livingstone.

Whiteford, G., Jones, K., Rahal, C. and Suleman, A. (2018). The participatory occupational justice framework as a tool for change: Three contrasting case narratives. *Journal of Occupational Science*, 25(4), pp. 497–508.

Whiteford, G. and Townsend, E. (2011). Participatory occupational justice framework (POJF 2010): Enabling occupational participation and inclusion. In F. Kronenberg, N. Pollard and D. Sakellariou (Eds.), *Occupational Therapies without Borders: Towards an Ecology of Occupation-Based Practices* (Vol. 2, pp. 65–84). Edinburgh, NY: Churchill Livingstone/Elsevier.

Wilcock, A. (1998). *An Occupational Perspective on Health*. Thorofare, NJ: Slack.

Index

For Product Safety Concerns and Information please contact our EU
representative GPSR@taylorandfrancis.com
Taylor & Francis Verlag GmbH, Kaufingerstraße 24, 80331 München, Germany

www.ingramcontent.com/pod-product-compliance
Lightning Source LLC
Chambersburg PA
CBHW060254220326
41598CB00027B/4095